03/14

HF

AGEING, HEALTHY AND IN CONTROL

FORTHCOMING TITLES

Psychology and Counselling for Health Professionals
Edited by Rowan Bayne and Paula Nicholson

Occupational Therapy for Orthopaedic Conditions
Dina Penrose

Teaching Students in Clinical Settings
Jackie Stengelhofen

Speech and Language Disorders in Children
Dilys A. Treharne

THERAPY IN PRACTICE SERIES

Edited by Jo Campling

This series of books is aimed at 'therapists' concerned with rehabilitation in a very broad sense. The intended audience particularly includes occupational therapists, physiotherapists and speech therapists, but many titles will also be of interest to nurses, psychologists, medical staff, social workers, teachers or volunteer workers. Some volumes are interdisciplinary, others are aimed at one particular profession. All titles will be comprehensive but concise, and practical but with due reference to relevant theory and evidence. They are not research monographs but focus on professional practice, and will be of value to both students and qualified personnel.

Ageing, Healthy and in Control

An alternative approach to maintaining the health of older people

STEVE SCRUTTON
BSc(Econ) MA CQSW DipEd

Social Work Manager, Northamptonshire Social Services Department, UK

CHAPMAN & HALL
London · Glasgow · New York · Tokyo · Melbourne · Madras

Published by Chapman & Hall, 2–6 Boundary Row, London SE1 8HN

Chapman & Hall, 2–6 Boundary Row, London SE1 8HN, UK

Blackie Academic & Professional, Wester Cleddens Road, Bishopbriggs, Glasgow GB64 2NZ, UK

Chapman & Hall, 29 West 35th Street, New York NY10001, USA

Chapman & Hall Japan, Thomson Publishing Japan, Hirakawacho Nemoto Building, 6F, 1–7–11 Hirakawa-cho, Chiyoda-ku, Tokyo 102, Japan

Chapman & Hall Australia, Thomas Nelson Australia, 102 Dodds Street, South Melbourne, Victoria 3205, Australia

Chapman & Hall India, R. Seshadri, 32 Second Main Road, CIT East, Madras 600 035, India

Distributed in the USA and Canada by Singular Publishing Group, Inc., 4284 41st Street, San Diego, California 92105

First edition 1992

© 1992 Steve Scrutton

Typeset in 10/12 Times by Mews Photosetting, Beckenham, Kent
Printed in Great Britain by St Edmundsbury Press, Bury St Edmunds, Suffolk

ISBN 0 412 38890 1   1 56593 032 0 (USA)

A catalogue record for this book is available from the British Library

Library of Congress Cataloging-in-Publication Data

Scrutton, Steve.
    Ageing, healthy, and in control : an alternative approach to maintaining the health of older people / Steve Scrutton. – 1st ed.
        p. cm. – (Therapy in practice series : 29)
    Includes bibliographical references and index.
    ISBN 1–56593–032–0
    1. Aged–Health and hygiene. 2. Aging. I. Title. II. Series.
RA564.8.S45   1992
613'.0438–dc20   92–21681
                                                            CIP

To my mother and in memory of my father

Contents

1

Nature and the importance of good health in old age

AGEING ...

Most people would like to live longer; but few wish to be older. Unfortunately, longevity results in old age. The paradox hinges on health. Whilst people want long life, they do not want to suffer from the pain, physical and mental decline and disease so often associated with ageing. For although ageing is not an illness, old age is too often seen as a losing struggle between health and disease.

All living organisms age, and within their allotted time-scales, die. The human body is made up of cells, each one a self-contained unit, but linked together in complex, interrelated structures, each with its own role to play within the body. Each cell contains 23 pairs of chromosomes, within which are the genes that form our genetic inheritance. Genes are made up of deoxyribonucleic acid, or DNA, the chemical which contains coded messages that form the basis of our individuality, instructing different parts of the cell machinery to perform in a particular manner.

DNA is being damaged throughout life, and reconstructed by enzymes which facilitate cell replacement and renewal. Longevity and the maintenance of health have been linked to the ability of the individual to repair his or her DNA. This function is believed to decline with age. As a result, there is a slowdown of physical functions, and an increase in physical vulnerability. Human ageing is associated with many factors, many of these the result of ill health, disease, or even genetic predisposition. The skin becomes wrinkled and blemished; there is greying and loss of hair; the bones become more brittle and more susceptible to fracture; and the joints wear and become painful. Muscle strength and co-ordination diminishes. The lungs become less elastic, making exertion more difficult; organ function deteriorates, with the heart, kidneys and liver becoming less efficient; the reproductive organs decline, along with the ability to procreate. The brain loses weight, memory weakens, and reaction times get slower. Eyesight and hearing deteriorates. There is a progressive decrease in resilience against illness and disease.

Nothing that lives can escape its own mortality: decline and death is a natural process that forms part of our total experience of life. Yet whilst ageing cannot be avoided, delaying the effects of ageing, and maintaining and extending youthfulness and fitness well into the ageing process, does seem possible.

In 1961, Hayflick and Moorehead showed that human cells only have a limited capacity to divide (Hunt, 1988). This limitation on the lifespan of human cells has been measured in cells taken from the brain, liver, muscle and skin, and no exception has been found to the general rule that normal cells cannot divide more than 50 times. Yet, whilst this would appear to rule out the idea of immortality, cells can live for much longer than the normal human lifespan. The cells of even the oldest surviving individuals can still undergo at least 20 more divisions.

Thus the paradox of wanting longer life without ageing can be seen more clearly. The mistake has been to measure life in terms of years, rather than in the quality of life possible in those years. In the past century, our fixation with extending life has seen the rise and fall of at least three highly publicized antiageing remedies – Bulgarian yoghurt at the end of the last century; sex gland transplants in the 1920s; and antireticular serum of the 1940s – all intent on extending rather than improving the quality of life.

Yet the desire is not to survive in poor and declining health, but to live retaining all the qualities associated with youth. Such an ideal is ultimately impossible, yet if youthfulness is defined as the absence of pain, discomfort, illness and disability, perhaps it is not quite so impossible. In a very real sense, individuals age to the extent that they acquire poor health, and they remain young to the extent that they maintain good health.

Chronological age, then, is not the most important indication of the ageing process. Age is more usefully measured in terms of the physical, mental and social functioning of the individual. The concept of functional, or biological age can be tested in a variety of ways, such as memory, hearing, vision, reaction times, lung function, and visual accommodation. These abilities give a better picture of the quality of life than can be judged by age alone. Any comparison made between older individuals at any age will show considerable differences in ability, functioning, health, and even life-expectancy.

Chronological age is at best only a rough indication of functional age. Because age norms imposed by society work to constrain behaviour, behaviour at a particular age cannot be assumed to be a reliable indication of the possibilities of that age. The present old as a class are clearly capable of much more than society allows them to express or experience, or than they allow themselves. Social roles in late life are ambiguously defined, so old age seems pointless, valueless. But it is known that deprived of specific roles, young people will respond the same as the old. In unemployment crises, for example, the young, rendered roleless, disengage, and become apathetic and indolent. Similar circumstances lead to similar responses irrespective of age. Many problems characteristic of the elderly are evoked by social conditions rather than innate processes.

(Walford, 1983)

The concept of functional age permits the development of certain understandings about ageing which are important to the developing argument contained herein:

- That to be old is not to be ill, or disabled.
- That old age and pain do not inevitably go together.
- That old age does not mean inevitable decline and decay.
- That even advanced old age is not a disease.

... HEALTHY ...

The maintenance of good health is crucially important to the quality of life in old age. Yet the maintenance of health is often obstructed by factors unrelated to chronological ageing. The health losses of old age are many and varied. Indeed, these losses can vary so much between ageing individuals that it is impossible to define ageing in any meaningful way. Yet despite this, a dominant social caricature emerges about the ageing process concerned with the progressive decline towards death, which is a potent mixture of fact, embellished with a considerable attachment of fiction.

The prospect of old age is widely feared. Yet it is not ageing itself that is feared, but the ageist stereotypes which associate it with pain, illness and disease. The close affiliation between the ageing process and dependency makes old age a sombre prospect and is so depressing that it can actually contribute to the very illness and dependency that are feared. Illness can threaten our quality of life and our very existence. For older people such fears represent a further burden on an already overburdened system. Fear exacerbates the physical symptoms of illness, and obstructs natural healing processes. Thus, when older people become ill, fear can arise by an inadequate understanding of the nature of the illness, what has caused it, and particularly its association with the ageing process.

A healthy approach to old age involves accepting the natural processes of ageing without unnecessary fears. There are three possible approaches to ageing. Pessimists compare themselves unfavourably with what they once were, considering themselves to be ill as a result of their age. Optimists will not consider themselves to be in anything but good health despite how they feel, unwilling to accept the normal deficits in the ageing process. The realist can more clearly perceive their deficits, whilst recognizing their potential regardless of how much or how little that might be.

The ageing individual should accept no more or less than that. No deficit is given or fixed at any particular age. An important objective in ageing should be to enjoy life fully, which means maintaining fitness and health, and youthful attitudes for as long as possible.

Yet whilst good health and happiness is best served by a positive acceptance of personal mortality, medical practice has had an unfortunate impact on health expectations in old age. On the one hand, medical knowledge has been increasingly reluctant to accept the inevitability of decline and death. The prospect of a replacement heart, or heroic treatment by wonder drugs or sophisticated machinery, has led to a growing and misguided denial of human mortality rather than accepting it as a normal part of life. Conversely, this medical optimism is applied mainly to younger people. Older people are often excluded, and more likely to be told that as they age they should expect to be ill more often, and more frequently in pain.

This combination of inappropriate medical aspiration, and age-related pessimism, serves only to contrast and heighten the fears and misconceptions about the nature of the ageing process. Medical ideas which deny the reality of ageing and death facilitate against the acceptance of reality. Ageism too readily permits the assumption that older people have to accept pain, illness and disease as an inevitable consequence of old age.

Too often, old people, their carers, and professional staff who should know better, do little that is constructive about major health issues relating to older people, dismissing the issues as the result of age rather than disease. To counteract this it is perhaps important to remember this maxim:

To be old and ill is as treatable as being young and ill.

... AND IN CONTROL

Illness in old age is feared because the relationship betweeen age and illness has been so widely misunderstood. Indeed, it can be said that many, if not most, older people do not understand illness at all. Doctors have become so influential and dominant in matters relating to health that they are assumed to have a monopoly of knowledge, and almost total responsibility for our health. Indeed, some medical propaganda would make it appear that older people owe their continuing existence to the skills of modern medicine.

The medical profession has probably assumed more responsibility for health than is 'healthy' for the individual. Many people have allowed medical professionals to assume complete responsibility for their health. The surfeit of professional advice, often allied with a paucity of discussion on health matters, can restrict many people from assuming personal control over their health.

Many writers have provided a critical analysis of the character of health and welfare services, these being seen to reinforce the dependency created through the wider social and economic system. It has also raised questions about the relationship of professionals to older people. How far do they challenge the low expectations that older people have about services? And to what extent do they contribute to the experience of old age as a period of dependency (Fennel *et al.*, 1988)? Older people find themselves treated and processed as commodities. Welfare services are criticized for stigmatizing older people, compounding their problems through the imposition of age-segregated policies. In practical terms, this analysis has raised issues about challenging the experience of older people as passive consumers of welfare and medical services.

What needs to be remembered is that doctors alone do not possess the gift of good health in old age. Indeed, the individual's best 'doctor' is often the individual, for within us all is the information about what is wrong, why it is wrong, and what can be done to put it right. Any diagnoses made by medical professionals are based primarily on the knowledge we give them, perhaps a form of knowledge which is underdeveloped, and based on skills which are underused. Yet such knowledge and skills do exist within each of us, however shrouded they have become by modern reliance on professional medical personnel.

Major developments during the past century, notably medical insurance schemes, including the National Health Service, have perpetuated one form of medical treatment: allopathic medicine. There are many forms of health care other than that available through your doctor or local hospital. Indeed, many alternative medical therapies can offer benefits for older people which remain largely unexplored. Moreover, there is nothing that modern medicine offers which cannot be questioned, challenged, and even refused. What is becoming increasingly evident is that modern medicine brings with it many inherent dangers, not least to older people. Indeed, older people more than most need to be warned.

Beware iatrogenic disease:
medicine itself can seriously damage your health

If the primary objective of the individual is to avoid premature ageing and death, to maintain health and the quality of life, the means to do so exists within each individual. Good health, in large measure, arises from a positive mental attitude and a sensible, healthy lifestyle. The problem is that whilst people are free to make themselves ill by their chosen lifestyle, they are not free, largely because of ignorance, to choose the method by which they can make themselves healthy. People need access to information, and to the great variety of medical knowledge and practice that is already in existence. When people have access to this information, personal fears begin to evaporate. Once the non-age factors which contribute to health are understood, then the destructive cycle of illness, fear and more illness can be broken, and the healing processes which exist within each individual can be set in motion.

This book seeks to develop a wider appreciation of health issues surrounding old age. It will attempt to remove the subject from the constraints imposed by conventional medical wisdom, and will challenge some dominant social attitudes which serve to restrict and disable older people. To achieve this, many widely held assumptions about the nature of old age, held by both young and old, and by professional and lay carers of older people, will be challenged. It will question the quality of health care that is provided for older people, particularly by dominant medical practice. As such, this may prove to be uncomfortable reading for those steeped in the conventional wisdom that modern medicine has a beneficial impact on the health and quality of life of older people.

By adopting a wider approach it is hoped that older people, and those who are responsible for aspects of their care, will be given an overview of the many and varied factors that can make up a programme designed to maintain health in old age.

The object throughout is to seek the extension of health rather than the extension of life. The aim of better health should not be to halt the ageing process, or even to delay death, for this raises false and unrealistic expectations. It is the quality, not the amount, of life that is important – maintaining the quality of life for as long into the ageing process as possible.

The fact and fiction that lies beneath the stereotypical caricature of ageing, and how best older people can maintain their health late into old age, is also examined. Every individual can moderate the effects of ageing, and this book sets out some ideas and materials which could contribute to this premise. Most of what needs to be done is under the control of the individual, who should be encouraged to seek his or her own way to a healthy old age. The choices to be made are known, and should be made as early as possible in his or her life. By making sensible and thoughtful choices, ageing people can live longer and, more important, live more fully without pain, illness and disease.

The message should be that it is possible to be ageing, healthy, and in control, an understanding which itself will help to assuage many fears about ageing.

2

Medical ageism: expectations of health in old age

All learning concerns the accumulation of knowledge and information. There is almost unquestioned acceptance that in most aspects of human life there is a state of constant progress, brought about largely by increased scientific knowledge.

Science has perpetuated the idea that it pursues its quest for knowledge impartially, giving the impression that it is based on principles that are entirely objective, and therefore unchallengeable. Through science, it is believed, humanity is becoming increasingly resourceful, ever more in control of its destiny, amd that such progress will continue alongside human capacity to learn. Increasingly since the eighteenth century there has been implicit faith in the power of science to solve problems, including the problem of disease.

What is not so often recognized is that human learning can also be thwarted by disinformation. Faulty and inaccurate knowledge can, and often does, prevent human progress. If Galileo had not helped us to 'unlearn' that the world was round, not flat, our knowledge of the universe would not have been possible. Despite our confidence in the state of current knowledge, we are as subject to misinformation now as at any time in the past. Moreover, the misinformation is as powerful in preventing progress and greater understanding as it has been in any past age.

The idea that scientific study, and the theories it has developed, are entirely 'objective' and dispassionate is not true. Science has often been used to confirm existing prejudice rather than to deny it. It has more frequently taken the side of powerful forces, explaining their status and influence, and justifying the comparative neglect of weaker social groups. Science has been used to justify the social inequalities of class, race and gender, and the oppression often based upon these grounds. It has been used to support and confirm supposed national and racial characteristics – the shiftlessness of blacks, and the disorderliness of Irish, the IQ of black people, and the prenatally determined psychological differences between men and women, for example. It has been used to explain power and status relationships, and the weakness and poverty that coexists in social life. In this way, science has often served to give credibility to existing social prejudice. Perhaps we should be far enough into the 'age of science' to see that scientific justification for our beliefs is, in many instances, entirely unreliable.

Too often, science prides itself with a sophistication its performance does not warrant. This is no more so than in medical affairs. Despite the writings of many critics of conventional medical performance (Dubos, 1959; Carlson, 1975; McKeown, 1979; and Illich, 1977), their message remains largely unknown to the vast majority of people. Knowledge, and the progress that can arise from it, has always been prevented by powerful social groups, whose ideas dominate what is to be believed, and not believed. Just as Galileo confronted a religious establishment which did not wish to examine the tenets of its time-honoured wisdom, these medical critics have been faced with a powerful medical establishment that has, thus far, successfully blocked any widespread discovery of the disinformation that exists within the field of medicine. The cassocks of the medieval Church have been replaced by the white coats of the conventional, allopathic medical establishment.

The influence of doctors is not restricted to medical matters. Their social role and status is now so strong that they have become firmly established as a vital part of conventional social wisdom, the dominant ideology which governs the way people think, believe and behave. They inform the attitudes of para-medical, and non-medical professional groups towards older clients, their capabilities, and their prospects.

Medical influence is no more apparent than in the health of older people. General attitudes and approaches to their health contain a major paradox. We are often told that people are living longer, and are healthier in old age than they have ever been. A large measure of credit for this is attributed to the skill and expertise of health services on the assumption that they have conquered or controlled the diseases which formerly would have killed old people. The response to such a claim is understandable; in the event of any illness or concern about an ageing individual, consider nothing else: just call the doctor.

Yet when the doctor is called, it is a common experience for older people to be told that their pain and illness are the inevitable consequence of ageing, and that there is little that can be done to

9

help them, a diagnosis usually unquestionably accepted because of the trust and respect that doctors have attained, especially with older generations.

Medicine seeks to sustain the positive view; but it is the negative perception which continues to prevail in practice, with ageing often seen as a disability or disease in its own right. Older people have become a category of patient, geriatrics, a distinct group whose illnesses are considered to be 'different', requiring separate study, and needing different treatment, a group to place alongside the physically and mentally disabled and the mentally ill as a special area of study.

The result is that the popular image of health in old age is one associated with an increase in pain, discomfort, illness, disease and dependence; loss of energy and personal drive; significantly greater need for rest; long and increasing periods of sickness; permanent experience of pain and discomfort; increasing immobility; the gradual loss of personal control and responsibility; the onset of incontinence, with resulting loss of dignity and self-respect; increasing confusion; and, ultimately, the most feared condition of all, senility.

This bleak picture of old age is universally powerful. Older people accept pain and discomfort as a normal and unavoidable feature of ageing. The widespread dread of ageing continues. Medical personnel usually confirm ageist perceptions through their diagnoses that illness is the natural, non-treatable consequence of ageing. Carers, and other professional staff involved in the care of older people, usually accept such explanations because they feel that it is beyond their area of competence to question medical opinions.

The truth of these contrasting perceptions of medical performance can be highly significant to the way old age is viewed. If it is true that medical expertise is extending life, and winning the battle of health in old age, the prospect of growing old should become progressively less daunting. Conversely, if we believe that living longer will bring with it the afflictions of pain, illness and disease that cannot be effectively treated, ageing will continue to attract a discouraging prognosis.

Negative medical practice needs to be challenged. The first step should be to examine general social attitudes about old age, and then to examine the performance of medicine itself. Medicine should no longer be allowed to make extravagant claims about its powers, whilst at the same time continuing to propagate negative ideas about ageing.

THE MYTH OF PHILANTHROPHY: THE SOCIAL CONSTRUCTION OF AGE

Age is one of the most important factors determining social status, changing as an individual is conceived, born, passes from babyhood to infancy, to childhood, to adulthood, and from thence to old age. Youth is identified with expectation and hope for what the future holds, both for the individual, and the society to which he or she belongs. Adulthood is a time of full vigour, strength and productivity, when the value of the individual is at its height.

Older people are frequently seen as a burden. The changes of status which occur as a result of these perceptions are determined by the dominant values and attitudes that exist within particular social groups at a particular time. Attitudes to older people are, in other words, socially constructed. The condition in which older people live is not, as is often assumed, an inherent or necessary part of 'being old'. This is demonstrated by the ways that each social group defines and reacts to older people, often in ways which are subtly, and sometimes fundamentally different to each other. Within each social group, certain key values and ideas tend to dominate the way people organize and make assumptions about the nature and experience of old age. These 'dominant' ideas usually reflect the interests of the most powerful, most influential social groups. They define, and then marginalize, older people by creating a set of negative values and attitudes which influence the way they are seen and, thereby, structure the way they lead their lives (Scrutton, 1990).

The dominant ideology that determines the status of older people in Western society is capitalism and, particularly, the importance attached to productivity. Work has moved to centre stage in several respects. It provides the economic basis for social functioning, and for political conflicts.

> Its impact goes far beyond simply assuring material survival or organizing political interests; it defines the cultural unity of modern Western societies as well as the identity of its members.,
>
> (Kohli, 1988)

The economic importance of productive work is perhaps the most obvious feature of the 'work society'. It provides people with their income, and also enables them to be consumers, these two factors together contributing powerfully to social status. But the work society has other important functions. It structures the way people lead their lives by integrating them into a pattern of social relations, providing the basis of day-to-day routine, and giving meaning and purpose to life by providing a feeling of usefulness and value.

The status of older people during the rigours of the agrarian and Industrial Revolution certainly declined. It was a time of ruthless exploitation of the weak by the strong, and older people, when their physical and mental powers declined, were no longer of primary economic importance. Many traditional community supports for older people were largely destroyed. Women, children and older people were expected to work long hours for subsistence wages, in dangerous and unhealthy factory conditions. Workers were squeezed for the last drop of production. It was a fierce, competitive world, in which there were few regulations to safeguard the rights of people forced to work within it.

The reaction to the worse excesses of this cruel system was nineteenth-century philanthropy, which attempted to improve the condition of older people who were, in many cases, being worked literally to their deaths. Retirement gradually became a legal obligation on employers, as did may other benefits of the welfare state.

> ... history, it is argued, has been the onward march toward citizenship, culminating in the mid-twentieth-century foundation of the welfare state. In our time, if elderly people have 'lost' their families, they have at least found a benevolent state to support them. We have moved, in this account, from welfare provided by the family to collectivist provision from state and society as a whole.
>
> (Fennel *et al.*, 1988)

Yet social philanthropy has had three unintended consequences. First, the unfortunate, if well-intentioned juxtaposition of exploitation and philanthropy has meant that older people, by virtue of compulsory retirement, have been made enforceably 'non-productive'. The withdrawal of work has meant that the main factor which contributes to social status is no longer available, the status of older people becoming the 'gift' of social philanthropy. The intended beneficiary of philanthropy, the ageing individual, has therefore suffered a significant loss. Retirement has forced older people into a position of financial dependence which allows them to be seen as a burden. Ambiguous attitudes towards the unemployed of all ages, a combination of contempt and sympathy, affects the way older people are seen, and see themselves. The unemployed have been regarded as inadequate, idle scroungers. The non-productive status of older people ensures that they are the recipients of social benefits, which many see as patronizing, undignified and debilitating. The problem with the 'philanthropy' offered to older people is that it is disabling, relegating them to the position of 'receiver' rather than 'provider'.

In this way, the low status of older people is not so much the result of the ageing process, but the structural conditions imposed upon them by disqualification from work – the key to social status.

The second consequence is that despite this disadvantage, which is usually unrecognized, older people are commonly believed to occupy a privileged position in modern society. The welfare state is seen as ample demonstration of a society which enables older people to live their final years in dignity, peace and tranquillity. This belief has arisen largely from a series of social and financial programmes, all genuine efforts to help older people escape the exploitation which followed the Industrial Revolution, namely, the development of pension schemes, universal health provision, social services, sheltered housing schemes, and residential care homes, all linked to 'the right' to retirement. Philanthropy has created the widely held belief that our dealings with older people are based on a compassionate, sensitive response to their needs, and a generous recognition and reward for their past services.

Yet the generosity of modern philanthropy has been questioned. Historians, such as Thomson (1984), has suggested that in the 1840–50s, about two-thirds of women aged 70 or more were in regular receipt of a Poor Law pension. Further, they have challenged current ideas concerning the generosity of modern provision in comparison with the past. Here, a crucial distinction is made between absolute and relative incomes. In terms of the former, pensions today can indeed provide a more prosperous standard of living. However, in a relative sense, payments in the last decades of the twentieth century are inferior to both the mid-nineteenth century and to Edwardian times.

> Elderly dependants from the 1830s to 1870s received from their communities cash allowances with value equivalent to two-thirds or more of the incomes of non-aged, working-class adults. It has been accepted in the present century (by contrast) that the elderly (in Britain) should be given little more than one-third of the resources of other adults.
>
> (Thompson, 1984)

Whilst this argument has been challenged (Hunt, 1990), the question of whether social provision is relatively greater or less than in previous centuries is finely balanced. Neither Thompson nor Hunt argues a case which supports the idea that older people are significantly better provided for today than they were in the supposedly 'bad old days' of the last century. Our philanthropy is, at best, paper thin in terms of the practical realities of being old in modern society. Certainly, the experience of being 'old' would suggest to many that social philanthropy is little more than an illusion, with the lives of many older people suggesting a harsher reality. Retirement pensions are fixed at subsistence levels, so that for most older people, the end of paid employment means a significant drop in income. Residential care for dependent older people is generally of a low standard.

The third consequence is that belief in social philanthropy lulls ageing people into a false sense of security. They are led to believe that they will be 'looked after' in their old age, and many will sit back expecting a better deal rather than actively demanding one for themselves. Nowhere does this apply more than in the area of health. Yet if the reality for older people is different to the rhetoric, why is this so? What social mechanism has consistently allowed the perceived, as opposed to the actual, treatment of older people to be so widely different?

AGEISM

Once social philanthropy towards older people has been challenged, some of the more difficult realities of old age can be examined. As has been said, we pay lip-service to idealized images of beloved, tranquil grandparents, wise, white-haired elders, but the dominant image disparages older people, and sees age as decay, decrepitude, and an undignified dependence.

The basis of social discrimination against older people lies within social values and attitudes. These are embedded within us all during the years of socialization. Thereafter, social discrimination is enshrined in the law, the operation of our institutions, and the activities of everyday life. Discriminatory practices against older people occur regularly each day, but pass largely unnoticed. These practices can be described under the broad term of ageism.

Ageism is the basis upon which older people, considered not as individuals, but as a homogeneous group, are discriminated against. It represents a set of widely held, or dominant prejudices about the nature, and experience of old age. They usually project negative, unpleasant images of older people which subtly undermine their sense of personal value and worth. Ageist assumptions restrict the social role and status of older people, structure the expectations that ageing people have about themselves, prevent them reaching their potential, and deny them equal opportunities. The result is the devaluing and disabling of older people, and the creation of the general aura of fear, dread, disgust and rejection that old age, and growing old, has assumed in our society.

(Scrutton, 1990)

Ageism is a form of power which denies individuality, grouping all older people together under crude stereotypes which both undermine and persecute them. Ageism exists within the minds of everyone, placed there by the powerful processes of socialization. Young infants do not discriminate on the basis of age. Their judgement of people is based entirely on whether they are treated gently or harshly, kindly or unkindly, or with love or disdain. Yet from the earliest years, young people are presented with unflattering images of old age, and it is this process of socialization that transforms ageing into something that is feared, and leads to the belief that older people are to be pitied or discounted.

Our educational system probably starts the process. There are many school textbooks, from the earliest reading stages, which portray older people as clumsy, frail, pathetic, needing to be helped across roads, whilst younger members of the family are happily enjoying an exciting and glamorous life. Many preschool poetry collections include material which present stereotypical pictures of older people (Tyler, 1986). These early influences are confirmed in later school years, not least in classic literature, where, for example, Shakespeare described old age as:

Second childishness, and mere oblivion, sans teeth, sans eyes, sans taste, sans everything.

(Shakespeare, As you Like It, Act 2)

Education also subtly confirms the ageist idea that older people are not educable, and not interested in personal development. Whilst educational legislation talks about the education of 'the people', it effectively caters for the education of children. Adults have no statutory rights to education, and as Tyler (1986) says:

. . . if adult education is marginalised then the education of older adults is marginalised to the margins of the margin.

The language we use is also ageist. Language is a powerful method of structuring attitudes about old age. Words and phrases in common usage, as well as definitions of age contained in classic English texts, such as *Roget's Thesaurus*, which seeks to arrange words 'according to the ideas which they express', describe old age in expressive, and almost invariable derogatory, infantalizing or pitying tones (Scrutton, 1990).

Sociological, psychological and religious ideas also reinforce stereotypical pictures of old age. The theory of disengagement (Chapter 6) has been an important sociological theory which discounted the needs of older people, as has the protestant work ethic (Weber, 1930), which, when linked with capitalist values, encouraged ideas that older people were less valuable. Social Darwinism is another, supposedly ethical, theory as it sought to give an explanation of evolution on scientific principles, which saw the survival of the fittest as a 'natural' mechanism. This mechanism has subsequently been used to explain and justify the continuing prosperity of the upper social classes, and the weeding out of the weaker members of species (Dubos, 1970), and can likewise be used to explain and justify ageism.

> We have, after all, an animal inheritance and it is animal instinct to challenge and destroy the leader of the herd when his strength begins to fail and to abandon to their fate animals which are too weak to keep up with the rest.
>
> (Norman, 1987)

The assumption that old people are rigid, less capable, less willing to adapt to new developments and unable to change, is firmly rooted in psychological theory. The father of modern psychology, Sigmund Freud (1905), was able to say that:

> ... psychiatry is not possible near or above the age of 50, the elasticity of the mental processes on which the treatment depends is as a rule lacking – old people are not educable.

This view continues to have an enduring effect on public perceptions of old age. The association between age, adaptability and psychological theory remains one of the major factors that disables older people, particularly within a society in which 'change' and 'progress' are becoming increasingly important.

Ageism is also deeply embedded in religious ideas. Our early Christian traditions have painted an unhappy portrait of old age, associating decrepitude, with all its ugliness, with the image of sin, and old age as as a curse and a punishment (Minois, 1989). All religion, not least Christianity, encourages the idea that our current condition is temporary, and certainly not as important as our place in the next life. Suffering is part of our preparation for the hereafter. Death, our link to a 'better' world, is to be welcomed rather than feared. Happiness, contentment, and fulfilment will be abundantly available in Heaven, Valhalla, or Nirvana. The idea that death is a happy release from old age both dismisses the importance of life for older people, and makes it a time to fear and dread. Conversely, the concept of Paradise is one of eternal youth, where the old are rejuvenated, where no one grows old, and where nobody dies.

These attitudes are important in shaping the expectations of older people. Their needs are discounted by theories that, at least implicitly, support the idea that older people are inherently less valuable, and less notable, than younger people. These views are internalized by ageing people, which in turn becomes important when attempts are made to justify the lack of social provision for older people, for older people themselves have low expectations.

MEDICAL AGEISM

Ageist ideas become embedded in the social structures which determine how older people are allowed, or permitted to live. Structural ageism is embedded into our laws and regulations involving employment, promotion and redundancy, retirement, welfare and pension rights, housing, and the care of dependent older people.

This can be clearly seen in the medical sphere. Medical opinion is an influential source of dominant social attitudes, inheriting from religion its role as the most powerful guardian of ageist ideology. Medical ideas are central to expectations about the 'normal' condition of older people. The image of old age as a time of pain, illness and disease is nurtured and encouraged by dominant medical opinion, which believes that illness is an unavoidable feature of normal ageing. The gradual deterioration of function is so widely expected that every decline tends to be attributed to age alone, even though disease produces similar results that can easily be mistaken with senescence.

The basis for medical ageism is a series of half-truths, untruths and over-generalizations about the biology of the ageing process, extended so that they appear to support explanations about the nature of life and health in old age that the facts do not support. Known aspects of the natural ageing process are removed from their context, and extended to produce explanations, or models of ageing, which are not supported or justified by the original premise. A few examples will indicate how this is achieved.

(a) Ageing is known to bring about a gradual decline in bodily functioning. Whilst this is generally true, the knowledge is often used to explain the inevitability of old age being linked with increasing physical and mental dependence. This is neither an inevitable, nor even a necessary consequence of ageing, and does not follow from the original premise.

(b) In old age there is greater susceptibility to illness and disease as the body loses its immunological protection, and suffers from a variety of wasting diseases. Yet this decline, which is usually a slow, imperceptible process, leads to the erroneous assumption that ageing and disease are so closely linked as to become synonymous. It becomes almost impossible to be both old and well.

(c) The gradual death of brain cells throughout life, believed to be irreplaceable, leads to an assumption that cell loss results in older people becoming less intelligent, less flexible, and less able to cope with the demands of a changing technological society. Yet the association between brain cell death and mental decline, forgetfulness, confusion, and ultimately dementia, has to be seriously questioned. The body produces 10 000 000 000 non-reproductive nerve cells, and normal loss throughout an entire lifetime is estimated to be only about 2.5%. Yet whilst this is not a significant factor in mental capacity, even in advanced old age, it does not prevent the belief that older people become less intelligent, or its widespread use to explain common errors, lapses in memory, and lack of motivation.

In these ways, medical ageism incorrectly associates illness in old age with the natural process of ageing. Once accepted as such, there is less reason to seek to cure it. The medical condition of older people can be considered as pre-ordained by age. Ageing, as an explanation for illness, does not allow a remedy. Illness, pain and disability becomes a natural and inevitable consequence of ageing that older people must accept. The result is that dominant social and medical attitudes expect older people to be ill, become dependent and to be a social burden. The only prospect for older people is further physical and mental decline, which they are expected to bear as an accepted, and acceptable part of the ageing process.

Yet medical ageism goes further. Conventional medicine dislikes death because it represents the ultimate failure. Yet as death is ultimately inevitable, older people seem only to confirm medical failure. The medical treatment of older people therefore receives low priority.

The fear of decline and death in old age arises largely from conventional medical thinking. There is a strong social taboo surrounding old age, death and decline. Simone de Beauvoir (1972) stated that:

> ... society looks upon old age as a kind of shameless secret
> that it is unseemly to mention.

The attitude of many health professionals is that major medical intervention with older people is not justified. Older people no longer have a significant social role, and are often seen to be doing little more than waiting for the 'release' of death. This further confirms the idea that illness in old age has to be accepted, that it is inevitably associated with old age, and that there is nothing that can be done.

The inaccuracy of medical ageism is embodied in those older people who retain their optimistic vision of life, affirming amid their losses and limitations that their existence is still good. They continue to learn and develop, to maintain their health, and their hopes for the future, thankful for what they can still accomplish. *Yet such optimism is possible for all ageing people.* As a well-known brandy advertisement says about 'the art of ageing gracefully':

> With age there comes maturity, character, clarity, taste and,
> finally, the proper degree of mellowness. Admirable qualities
> all, in Man as well as ...

If this was generally perceived to be the outlook for older people, it would herald a more prosperous deal for them. Unfortunately, such perceptions are the exception rather than the rule. Many older people are unable to maintain sufficient optimism and energy to resist ageist attitudes. They internalize ageist views about their own health, accepting that the best is behind them, with the worst aspects of decrepit old age yet to come. The result is that most older people, and their carers, take a passive approach to ageing health, discounting suggestions to investigate and treat the causes of illness.

THE PSYCHOLOGY OF AGEISM: THE IMPACT ON OLDER PEOPLE
. . .

The internalization by older people of the bleak outlook of ageism leads to the underlying assumptions becoming self-fulfilling prophecies. The dominant social, economic and medical description of old age is accepted by older people, who soon expect no more from their life than the description offers. It limits what older people expect of themselves, what they feel they can, and are expected to do; it becomes part of their reality. The consequence is that older people live in a way which confirms and perpetuates ageist stereotypes. Older people *do* disengage from social life, they *do* accept lower social status, they *do* adapt to their lack of social role. Eventually, they *do* readily accept illness and disease, and they *do* wait despondently for decline and death.

Ageism makes invalids of people on the basis of age. Older people seen as invalids are discouraged from work, exercise or endeavour. The practice of 'caring' for older people often assumes responsibility for activities and responsibilities that they should retain for themselves, making them prematurely dependent. All this makes both the prospect and reality of old age worse than it should be. Not only do older people receive poorer social, economic and medical consideration, they actually accept that this is right and just.

Invalidism leads to boredom, loneliness, confinement, and often therafter, to hypochondria. Medical perspectives of older people as 'sick', do not, in themselves, make them sick or idle, but it provides a powerful rationale against allowing older people to act in any other way. It is essentially medical arguments which suggest to older people that they should not work, should not exercise, and are not sufficiently flexible to take a full part in social life.

It is this ageist circularity which undermines the prospect and experience of old age. Dominant ideology is powerful. It pervades the thinking and the expectations of both young and old. It is not sufficient to point out that older people get a bad deal; it is essential that the underlying ideological assumptions which support and justify the deal are questioned and tackled before significant change will occur.

Eventually, everyone has to recognize that with ageing there will be a slowing down in functioning. Biology should not be the issue for older people, for it can be accepted. It is ageism, the power struggle with younger people, which disqualifies, discounts and invalidates.

. . . AND THEIR CARERS

Ageism discounts the personal strengths and retained capabilities of older people. The carers of older people, whose motivation and commitment need not be questioned, are no less susceptible to the process. Their caring task necessitates working with the more dependent older people, rarely seeing fitter, more independent people who do not conform to the stereotypical picture. Consequently, their work can reinforce, on a daily basis, popular ageist stereotypes of the nature of old age.

Moreover, the nature of the caring task can sometimes shield carers from what they are doing for others. They 'do things' for older people because they assume that this, by its very nature, is caring. Carers can easily confirm elderly invalidism by making older people dependent upon their care. Older people cannot be expected to do things, so carers, as caring people, will do it for them. The more that doctors treat, and social workers care, the more they are called to do so, and the more indispensable they become. The debilitating nature of removing personal responsibility from the individual is usually rarely considered, but older people can be placed in the 'sick role' by caring. Invalidism makes older people seem dependent upon carers for their physical survival; this is often what is experienced by many older people, and how they are seen by their carers, and by professional staff.

The stereotypical picture of health in old age does exist, and can be seen in the lives of countless thousands of older people. What needs to be challenged is the social creation of false images of life in old age and their too ready acceptance by older and younger people alike. Professional carers have to decide what basis in reality the ageist health stereotypes have, for it is important to prevent them from becoming self-fulfilling. If professional care staff continue to have low expectations of health in old age, and if this expectation is based in ageism rather than the biological process of ageing, it will continue to undermine what older people are able to do and achieve for themselves.

More important, ageing individuals need to consider what they can do to remain fit and healthy for as long as possible, once removed from these socially constructed restraints.

Ageism is used to confirm the low priority given to older people, and to justify the low standards of care they receive. Improved priorities and standards of care for older people are involved in tackling the underlying discrimination that older people face, and this is based in social attitudes.

Yet it follows that if dominant social ideas structure the way older people are treated, it is possible to vary them. Social attitudes towards age are not the natural and unavoidable consequence of the ageing process. Age status varies between generations, and between cultures, so it is possible to reconstruct social perceptions of older people, and the nature of old age. Yet this will only happen when older people, and their carers, begin to consider the impact of ageism that more comprehensive strategies towards the health of older people will be constructed.

3

Allopathic medicine:
the medicalization of old age

Throughout the developed world, medical practice is dominated by a single form of medicine. For most people, going to a doctor, or hospital, means receiving allopathic medical treatment. Allopathy is a system of medicine which treats disease by inducing an opposite or contrary condition. Thus, to cure constipation, the patient is administered medication that would normally induce diarrhoea; likewise, for fever, drugs which reduce temperature are used. It delivers medical treatment in two major ways: the administration of drugs which work on the biochemistry of the 'problem' part, or by direct surgery, involving its modification, removal, or replacement, often using complex techniques, and advanced technological equipment.

Indeed, allopathy has been involved in the search for 'heroic' treatments for illness and disease through the development of many complex techniques and procedures, often to the exclusion of simpler procedures favoured by traditional forms of medical practice. It tends to prefer the spectacular feats of organ transplantation to the mundane task of treating arthritis.

The dominance of allopathy is a major change from the situation which existed during the early nineteenth century, and before, when allopathic medicine had an appalling reputation. The status of doctors was low, and a visit something to be avoided, even if it could be afforded. This cynicism was well founded given the methods employed, which included bleeding, violent purges, and heavy doses of toxic mercury-based drugs. Surgery prior to anaesthetics, antibiotics and efficient hygiene, was also a highly risky venture (Griggs, 1981).

More traditional forms of medicine, based on time-honoured empiricism, were favoured. Traditional health care attributed considerable importance to the inherited wisdom of community elders, usually female, consisting of treatments based upon local plants and herbs, practised with a blend of art, magic and superstition, but supported by centuries of practical knowledge and experience. The Industrial Revolution profoundly affected these rural, community-based medicines. The population moved to the towns; herbal medicine remained in the countryside.

Life expectancy in the newly urbanized, industrialized towns was low, and infant mortality was high. Epidemics killed thousands of people each year, often devastating entire communities with apparently little hope or expectation of cure. Yet by the beginning of the twentieth century, the situation had been radically changed, apparently brought about by allopathic medicine. Killer diseases, such as smallpox, typhoid, cholera and tuberculosis, seemed to be under control, life expectancy had improved, and young children stood a better chance of living to adulthood. The success was attributed to the introduction of new drugs and new surgical techniques, particularly during the last century.

The 'new' medicine soon won political support in the form of medical insurance schemes, ensuring that everyone was able to benefit from the new science. This further reinforced the dominance of allopathy by giving people immediate access to just one form of medical care. The National Health Service, established in 1948, brought allopathic medical practice to everyone, regardless of income. Hopes were high. Whilst there might be a 'backlog' of work arising from those people who had hitherto not been able to afford treatment, after these initital demands had been met it was confidently expected that national health standards would improve, and that demand for health services would decrease.

For these reasons, society has placed increasing reliance upon the allopathic medical profession, who, in turn, have been successful in persuading people that they, and they alone, should be responsible for the prevention and treatment of illness. Other forms of medicine, such as homeopathy, naturopathy, and herbalism, which formerly had strong followings, have been progressively marginalized, eventually becoming fringe activities undertaken only by a few people in isolation to mainstream medicine.

The last century witnessed considerable allopathic medical achievement which sustains this confidence. The disease pattern has been radically altered. Infectious disease is no longer the primary cause of death. The success attributed to medicine in fighting diseases such as diptheria, tuberculosis, polio, pneumonia, syphilis, tetanus, scarlet fever, measles, and rickets, has led to an increase in medical status, the assumption being that the 'new' medicine, firmly based on scientific principles, has successfully freed humanity from the ignorance and superstition of traditional forms of medicine, and from former killer diseases.

Medical science has also led to a considerable advance in understanding the intricate workings of the body, and this has proven operationally useful. It has helped scientists to delineate more precisely the scope of their investigations, instead of attempting to understand the body as a whole. It has enabled the discovery of the chromosome, the gene and DNA, the germ and the virus, all of which formed the basis for the development of new treatments for illness.

Emergency treatment has assisted in dealing with accidents and other acute emergencies. Modern anaesthesia enables longer and more complex operations to be carried out on people of all ages, during which the heart and lungs can be sustained, and bodily functions monitored more accurately. Many operations can restore normal health from disabling and life-threatening conditions. Kidney dialysis maintains life, and kidney transplants extend life for many who would otherwise die. Hormone replacement therapy is now successful in treating glands controlling the metabolism, growth and sex hormones. Thyroid problems can now be better controlled by hormone treatment. Diabetes can be stabilized, although not cured, by insulin treatment. Hip replacement operations can give many years of mobility to older people who would otherwise become housebound and in permanent pain. The removal of cataracts can restore sight.

Drug development has played an important role. The development of sulphonamide in the 1930s, and penicillin in the 1940s, gave medicine greatly improved powers to control infection. It has been claimed that antibiotics have halved the number of deaths which might otherwise have been expected, and has reduced the lethal impact of a whole range of other diseases.

Overall, there is widespread confidence that what allopathic medicine does not know today will eventually be learnt, and that current areas of medical failure can be explained by past inadequacies, now resolved, or attributed to isolated problems which were not inherently part of general medical practice. The only consistent complaint concerning medicine appears to be that it receives insufficient resources.

Yet the more sanguine hopes and expectations for allopathic medicine have not been realized. Current medical influence is based on its past effectiveness in conquering infectious killer disease, and the promises it makes about its ability to deal with modern illness.

Both claims need to be carfully examined, for if medical performance matched the many claims made for it, continued support would be justified. However, there is considerable evidence to the contrary.

Claims about the past effectiveness of allopathic medicine are probably an exaggeration. There is well-supported evidence that major reductions in tuberculosis, bronchitis, pneumonia, influenza, cholera, diarrhoea, dysentery, typhoid, scarlet fever and diphtheria, all took place before the introduction of the modern treatments which have been attributed with their demise. Prior to the introduction of streptomycin, the death rate from tuberculosis had fallen to one-tenth the rate 100 years earlier. Typhoid died out in Britain before the development of any form of medical treatment. Ninety-five per cent of the reduction in death rate from cholera occurred before the introduction of intravenous treatment in the 1930s. The death rate from bronchitis, pneumonia and influenza had been falling steadily since the early twentieth century, and the introduction of antibiotics has not speeded up the process (Illich, 1979). The impact of better social conditions, improved sanitation and nutrition were all more significant than is popularly credited, although this is now acknowledged in most medical texts.

As far as modern claims are concerned there is now evidence indicating that health is declining, that morbidity and mortality scales have reached a plateau, that life-expectancy is beginning to tail off, and might be falling. Rather than dying from traditional killer diseases, people are instead dying of diseases, such as coronary thrombosis, which were virtually unknown to nineteenth-century physicians. The devastating epidemics of infectious disease, such as typhoid, tuberculosis, cholera and smallpox, have been replaced by equally devastating epidemics of strokes, high blood pressure, heart attacks, behavioural disorders, allergies and degenerative diseases, leaving us little healthier than we were 100 years ago (Mackarness, 1976).

Perhaps more important for the quality of life of older people is the increasing incidence of many chronic, crippling diseases, with little evidence that medical science has any solution for them. These are not attractive areas of medical practice. Allopathy concentrates on areas of conspicuous therapy, and heroic intervention, where large salaries and international reputations can be won. The result is that whilst hearts and lungs can be transplanted, arthritis continues to undermine quality of life of many older people. This invites many important questions. Why, in spite of unprecedented technological progress, and the expenditure of vast sums of money, does good health continue to elude us, especially in our later years?

And why is medicine still unable to explain many modern ailments, or discover effective remedies?

The cost of medicine has rocketed. Health care is consuming an ever-increasing percentage of national income, yet despite this massive resource commitment, medicine cannot demonstrate to health economists that higher spending is leading to improved health. The medical establishment has come under increasing pressure to demonstrate that increased spending brings tangible benefits in terms of improved health. Indeed, there is growing political recognition that expenditure is not resulting in significantly improved treatment of modern diseases, lower mortality rates, or increased life expectancy, although the connection being made focuses on funding and expenditure rather than questioning medical efficiency.

This is happening, however, in the poorer, Third World nations, who are increasingly wary of adopting similar health care systems, and supported by the World Health Organization, are making a closer examination of the relationship between health spending and health. The tendency is to place increasing emphasis on the need for a broader approach to health care, relying on simpler, less technical, and cheaper forms of treatment.

The idea that allopathic medicine is, by definition, 'good' began to be re-examined in the 1950s. Dubos (1959), a member of the orthodox medical fraternity, pointed out that the achievements of medical science were less spectacular than were being claimed. Cochrane (1972) found that the work of doctors and hospitals could not be shown to contribute significantly to the outcome for the patient. Carlson (1975) studied the impact of medical care on people's lives, and produced evidence which suggested that it had little to do with any broader definition of health, which concerned itself with the maintenance of health rather than the treatment of disease. McKeown (1979) examined a number of diseases, considered the contribution made by medicine, and concluded that it made only a relatively small contribution. Illich (1977), who surveyed the historical evidence, came to the conclusion that 'medical intervention has made, and can be expected to make, a relatively small contribution to the prevention of sickness and death'.

It is important that these claims are examined, for if they are justified, the domination of allopathic medicine must be seriously questioned. Unfortunately, it is extremely difficult to do so. The powerful professional and commercial medical establishments, supported by a vast medical bureaucracy, have a vested interest in the maintenance of allopathic medicine. Powerful medical interests have prevented the critique of modern medicine from reaching a wider audience by their control of medical knowledge, and the funds available to finance both medical intervention, research and publicity. Information is power, and conventional medicine controls the information on which health decisions are made. Allopathy seeks to safeguard its dominant position, and resist challenges about the quality and value of what it offers. The public receives its information from a media which perpetuates the view that allopathic medicine is winning the battle against disease, and steadily improving standards of national health care.

Faith in allopathic health care therefore remains strong. The public continues to believe that medicine produces health, as witnessed by public demands for increased funding, and local charitable efforts to equip hospitals with the latest medical gadgetry. The questioning of medical orthodoxy, where it exists at all, comes from a small, disregarded minority. Indeed, to many people brought up on a diet of conventional medical wisdom, contrary ideas can seem deeply alarming.

Despite this, with the ever-increasing demands on health services, and their ever-burgeoning costs, a reassessment of the worth of allopathic medicine is under way. There are a number of major criticisms that need to be outlined, all focusing on the treatment of disease through the elimination of symptoms rather than dealing with the wider, underlying causes of disease and ill-health. Allopathy is based on three fundamental premises: first that diseases are specific entities, whose symptoms can be dealt with by specific interventions that relate to them; second, that the human body is a machine, each one essentially alike, so that patients with similar symptoms can be treated with similar methods; and third, that health is the product of medical care services, specific to the disease (Carlson, 1975).

Allopathic medicine constrained by scientific method, searches for single causes, usually in isolation, thereby tending to oversimplify the causation of illness. It suggests that illness strikes at random, arising primarily at the level of cell chemistry or microbiology. Although medicine does acknowledge wider social and emotional influences on health, the explanations it favours remain essentially at this level, with disease being explained as a malfunction within the body, and the solution resting in tinkering with internal biology.

This has led to the allopathic tendency of interpreting health as a battle by medical staff against a malfunctioning biology, a battle scenario enhanced by interpreting illness as discrete diseases, with specific origins, names and treatments. Whilst it is useful to have a system for classifying symptoms and causes, for medicine the specification of discrete disease entities have another significance. They represent a diagnosis, which, in turn, implies a knowledge of causation, and thus an indication of possible cure. This functional, or reductionist, view of the natural world, the belief that an effective understanding of the complex human organism can be achieved by investigating the properties of isolated parts, is a major criticism of allopathy. Naming the disease without an ability to cure does not assist the patient. Moreover, many so-called 'disease' entities, sounding ever more complex, are often no more than names for a collection of symptoms, without known cause or cure, such as 'non-specific urethritis', or 'irritable bowel syndrome'.

The pursuit of a single, biological cause for discrete illnesses is bolstered by medical organization, with its highly specialist structure. Illness is localized within these restricted systems, which have become an increasingly solid structural barrier to seeing whole bodies, and whole people. This in turn has led to a trend away from concern for the individual towards a more impersonal approach to the problems of disease. Medical treatment pays attention to the 'parts', or to disease processes. This 'engineering' approach has led to analogies between the delivery of health services, and the repair of motor cars. The 'sick' car is examined by mechanics, and the faulty parts located, repaired or replaced. The factors which have led to the fault are rarely examined, nor is the damage that might have occurred to other peripheral parts. Once the immediate fault is corrected the car functions again until the next link in the network begins to fail. Thunhurst (1982) has likened this process to the treatment received by the casualties of a hazardous social system, who have their defective parts patched up, only to be returned to the same social environment which contributed to the initial problem.

The result is that allopathy tends to concentrate on the individual as a 'machine', concerned with the mechanical structure and functions of the body, and with specific disease processes. Initially, medicine studied the 'body-machine', measuring the structure and functions of the mechanical aspects of the body. During the nineteenth and twentieth centuries, the emphasis shifted to chemical interpretation of living processes. The resulting tendency has been to study and treat individual parts of the body in isolation to the whole person, and as medical knowledge increases, it is specializing within ever narrower aspects of the human organism.

Yet medical answers are not emerging by looking ever deeper inside the organism; allopathic medicine has rarely identified the ultimate cause of illness. The ongoing search for causation ever deeper into body chemistry continues, yet even when a gene, germ, virus, hormone, or enzyme is implicated, it rarely leads to more effective treatment. Certainly, 'reductionist' research has failed to make significant headway with many of the modern diseases of ageing. Whilst such knowledge may be valuable, delving into the intricacies of the human organism has missed the essential wholeness of the human organism, within which no single part, however vital, can function properly without relating to other parts, however seemingly trivial.

This is no more evident than in the separation of mind and body, which many medical scientists believe is leading medicine into a blind alley precisely because the philosophical ideas on which it is based are unsound. Descartes taught that the body was a machine whose structure and operation fall within the province of human knowledge, whilst the study of the mind did not. This approach has led allopathic medicine to neglect questions about the mind and emotions, to concentrate instead on the simpler, more tangible problems of the body, to which the knowledge of physics and chemistry can be more directly applied.

The self-imposed limitations of Cartesian dualism has resulted in medicine tending to study man as a non-thinking, non-feeling entity (Dubos, 1970). Reductionist methodology, which characterizes most modern research and treatment, interprets disease as an isolated malfunction rather than part of a wider, more complex process. As a result, treatment has tended to become depersonalized, with individuals feeling less involved in what is happening to their bodies. Many people find the increasing impersonalization of medical treatment difficult to accept; even the family doctor is increasingly seen as an extension of medical machinery.

There is increasing evidence that looking outside the body may produce more clues about the cause of illness. Many chronic health conditions are being linked to pollution, and the stresses of modern life. Allopathic medicine has tended to neglect the social and emotional processes which contribute to health. Indeed, it has increasingly missed the literal meaning of the word *health*, for 'to heal' means 'to make whole'.

Nor does allopathic medicine appear to base its view of illness and disease on any clear scientific rules or principles, or demonstrate in practice a consistent overall approach to either diagnosis or treatment. It places considerable reliance upon 'trial and error' which has led to the fashionable treatments of one period being replaced in the next by something quite different. Blood-letting and leeching were the chief therapeutic techniques of the nineteenth century, these being gradually replaced by highly toxic chemical drugs, and by surgical techniques. A later generation of treatment using vaccine and serum then became popular. More recently, this uncertainty of approach is regularly compounded by the introduction of new 'miracle' drugs, followed by their withdrawal following revelations concerning their dangers to health. This leads, perhaps, to the most serious criticism of allopathic medicine, and one which is leading to most public concern.

IATROGENIC DISEASE

The reliance placed on allopathic medicine becomes more serious when iatrogenic, or 'doctor induced' illness is considered. Iatrogenic disease results directly from medical or surgical treatment. It is not a new idea. Moliere, Tolstoy and Shaw all claimed that the average individual would be better off without doctors. Confidence in the doctor is a relatively new phenomenon, overcoming a long-standing cynicism about allopathic approaches to health.

It is the scientific nature of allopathy that is claimed to make it preferable to other forms of medical treatment. The aim of scientific investigation is to systematically isolate relevant factors, and to test the effects of these factors under objective, repeatable conditions in order to judge the soundness of the conclusions. Yet when allopathic medical practice is examined, its 'scientific' base has to be seriously questioned. New drugs discovered this century appeared to produce such miraculous results that the public became conditioned to accept their value, without considering their side-effects. Following the thalidomide tragedy of the early 1960s, evidence has accumulated suggesting that many medical techniques and products, including many of the most commonly used, have little or no efficacy. Moreover, there is now considerable evidence that allopathic medicine can be positively dangerous to health. Many forms of treatment, introduced initially as miracle cures, and some used for many years, have been withdrawn when subsequently found to have harmful, often lethal side-effects.

Whilst drugs, such as antibiotics, have contributed to life expectancy by reducing deaths previously caused by killer infectious diseases, they have not been as successful, or as central, to the trend as generally believed. Some drugs have certainly proved their worth in restricted circumstances, but without exception, their toxic side-effects are causing increasing concern, and have raised many questions. Is modern medicine 'scientific ' for ensuring the safety

31

of clinically tested toxic drugs? Or for proving beyond question the value of surgical procedures and medical machinery?

Some criticism of allopathic practice has been totally condemnatory. Illich (1977), in a major exposition of iatrogenesis, described the medical establishment as a 'major threat to health'. Inglis and West (1983) doubt that allopathic medicine is capable of changing:

> The bleak fact is that the profession as it stands cannot change
> its ways, certainly not fast enough to meet the public's need.

Under the heading of clinical iatrogenesis, Illich (1977) described the physical damage caused by medical treatment, including the unwanted side-effects of scientifically tested and medically approved drugs. Whilst allopathic drugs have always been potentially poisonous, their iatrogenic effects have increased with their complexity and widespread use. People suffer because they take the wrong drug, or too much of it, or in dangerous combinations with other drugs. Drugs might prove effective for the conditions they treat, but cause damage in other areas of the body, or weaken the body's natural resistance to illness. Some drugs become addictive, others mutilate, whilst others are mutagenic. Indeed, drug side-effects have become so common that Hurwitz and Wade (1969) calculated that one-tenth of all hospital admissions were the result of prescribed drugs, whilst Williamson and Chopin (1980) found adverse drug reactions in 15.3% of prescribed drug takers.

Even apparently successful drugs, still widely believed to be beneficial to health, are now implicated in iatrogenesis. Drugs administered to arthritics to relieve pain were actually hastening the destruction of their joints (Hope, 1989). Antibiotics have greatly enhanced the treatment of bacterial infections, killing many organisms defined as harmful. In doing so, they provide effective protection from many severe, potentially deadly diseases. Yet their use has become widespread and indiscriminate. They do not prevent the return of infections, to which many older people are prone, and there is evidence that they may make recurrence more likely. They can also cause other problems, such as thrush and diarrhoea; their over-use can hasten the development of bacteria resistant to antibiotics, and as antibiotics artificially recreate natural functions of the body, they can depress the body's fight against disease, and gradually weaken natural immune defence mechanisms, and inhibit the development of the body's own resistance. Mansfield (1988) warned that we should 'look at antibiotics as a precious capital reserve, to be drawn on a few times only in your life, if at all'. Cannon (1989) traced the origins of his wife's colon cancer to the overuse of antibiotics, which are known to have side-effects on the digestive system, which occur when antibiotics kill natural organisms required for the proper digestion of food.

Surgical operations can also form part of clinical iatrogenesis, with problems arising through negligence, incompetence, callousness or malpractice. Some techniques, such as coronary bypass surgery, have been introduced before there were adequate trials testing their efficacy. Overall, there appear to be few rules or guidelines for surgical intervention, and many studies of the geographical variations in the rate of surgery have shown striking differences. These indicate that many standard operations, such as tonsillectomy, appendicectomy, hysterectomy and mastectomy, are performed quite unnecessarily. Moreover, the performance of many serious or complex operations have little proven value in extending life expectancy, or improving quality of life.

Infection caught whilst in hospital, particularly when recovering from an operation, is another problem, especially serious at a time when the body's ability to cope with the germs that abound within hospital environments is low, and doubly so since many of the causative organisms are now often resistant to antibiotics.

Social iatrogenesis follows clinical iatrogenesis (Illich, 1977), arising when addiction or dependence on medical care develops. This deprives individuals of the belief that they can exercise control over their health. Medical intervention is too often seen as the only solution to health and, indeed, to many other problems that people face. Sick people are encouraged to become consumers, not least because the prescription of drugs, and the performance of operations, are the basis of both professional reimbursement, and industrial profit. The over-consumption of drugs, even perhaps prescribed drug addiction, is thus socially sanctioned.

The impact of iatrogenesis on older people is particularly striking. The practice of medicine, upon which many older people place their trust, can contribute to their sickness. Indeed, the unquestioning faith that many older people have in medicine can actually lead to an increased susceptibility to iatrogenic disease.

The physiological changes of ageing makes older people particularly prone to adverse drug side-effects, this vulnerability arising from several factors, of which three are most important.

a) Ageist medical practice often means that drugs are prescribed on the basis that 'nothing else can be done'. It is well documented that errors in medication occur more frequently than commonly realized or admitted.

b) Poly-pharmacy is a particular problem for older people. There is a tendency for doctors to over-medicate, and then fail to maintain the necessary vigilance in prescribing drugs beyond the point that their use was indicated, or in combinations that are safe. This often results in creating health problems more severe than those for which the medication was originally prescribed.

c) Reduced kidney and liver function makes it more difficult for the older body to remove toxic substances, to effectively obtain energy and manage energy reserves, or to maintain adequate immune defence. Drugs take longer to clear from the system. The functioning of many organ systems become reduced, so the body becomes more susceptible to illness and other debilitating conditions, often with life-threatening consequences.

Benzodiazepine drugs, regularly prescribed for older people, can serve as an example of the iatrogenic effects of modern drugs. Commonly known as Valium, Librium and Mogadon, they calm the mind, relax muscles, induce sleep, and have been widely used to treat depressive illnesses. Indeed, they have often been considered a general panacea for the stresses and anxieties of life. Since their introduction in the 1950s, they have been considered entirely safe, with even an overdose apparently leading to little more than drowsiness. However, the benzodiazepines are now known to have harmful effects when used regularly for more than a few weeks. These effects are most marked with older people, for they are eliminated from the body slowly, with accumulations causing drowsiness, lack of co-ordination, and so increasing susceptibility to falls and fractures.

One benzodiazepine has now been withdrawn following many years of doubt and concern. Halcion, widely used for insomnia, has been found to cause nightmares, aggression, suicidal tendencies, paranoia, and hallucinations (Panorama, BBC Television, 14 October 1991). The programme described the falsification, even the faking, of clinical trials, the suppression of information, and even lying by the drug company concerned. What was not mentioned in the programme was that the drug was widely used with older people; it was described in the British National Formulary as 'useful in the elderly'.

The benzodiazepines are often prescribed to deal with the extremes of feeling which are engendered by the stresses of life. Yet mood-altering medication cannot change the reality of life, but merely give a temporary feeling that matters are better. Moreover, by suppressing normal social restraints they can provoke uncharacteristic outbursts of antisocial behaviour, often involving aggression and violence. They are now known to cause impairment of memory and concentration, depression, and ultimately, brain damage and confusion.

Moreover, their immediate effectiveness in relieving symptoms, such as anxiety and insomnia, often encourages their continuing use, leading to tolerance, dependence and withdrawal symptoms. Tolerance makes the drug less effective, so a greater quantity is required. In time, the drug becomes indispensable, and users become dependent. Many older people soon require the drug for psychological and physical reasons, often quite different to those for which they were originally prescribed.

The more serious the diagnosis, and the more dire the prognosis, the more careful the older individual should be about the prescription of allopathic medication. The restraints on using more powerful, more toxic drugs are progressively reduced in proportion to the increasing serious of the illness. This, too, often makes older people more likely to be prescribed powerful, toxic drugs in response to declining health, their side-effects ensuring a downward spiral of ill-health, increased medication, and more serious illness. More detailed references to the side-effects of drugs, and their specific impact on older people, are described in a useful guide published by Age Concern England (Blair, 1985).

THE MEDICALIZATION OF SOCIAL LIFE

The medical establishment has become an extremely powerful and influential social force. The doctor occupies a position of the highest professional status. Medicine has established the principle that clinical judgement is unquestionable, a powerful notion that dominates many areas of health service activity. Moreover, unlike other professional groups, doctors occupy a leading role in the infrastructure of medical management. This means not only that they have complete clinical autonomy, but power to control many aspects of service delivery. Recent changes in the management structure of the NHS does not fundamentally alter this situation.

Doctors are not the only representatives of medical power. The pharmaceutical industry has a dominant and influential position; it is the drugs they produce which allopathic medicine depends upon.

Drug manufacture is highly lucrative. The market is controlled by a few multinational companies. Their profits are based upon business practices with which the medical profession colludes, including monopoly pricing which allows massive price mark-ups, and patenting legislation which protects against competition. The companies sell to a limited number of medical practitioners, who are encouraged to prescribe their products by a variety of promotional activities.

The industry that supplies medical instruments and equipment operates similarly. Conventional medicine is increasingly reliant on expensive, highly complex technology, the production of which is dominated by a few multinational companies. Body scanners, incubators, renal dialysis units, respirators, laboratories and operating theatres, are marketed as essential, urgently required, 'life-saving' equipment. The performance of this equipment, when studied closely, rarely matches up to the claims or, indeed, to their high cost. The use of many thousands of tests, from simple blood tests, to X-rays, nuclear magnetic resonance scans, electrocardiograms, intensive care units, and many others, have proven to be costly for the health services, and misleading, time consuming, painful, and even dangerous for the patient (Thunhurst, 1982).

The widespread acceptance of medical power has led to many natural functions being taken over, or medicalized. Pregnancy and childbirth is an example of this process, highlighted by the women's movement. Although this is normally a natural, trouble-free process, modern medicine has made it a complicated process, dominated by medical supervision. Hospital admissions are the rule, with induced births, and an increasing number of Caesarean sections. Many women find that giving birth has become a technical process of which they are no longer in control, and many women are now questioning whether hospital births are safer than home births, particularly when the dangers of hospital infection are taken into account.

Yet the medicalization of health is particularly apparent in old age, with debilitating results for many older people. Medical propaganda influences all age-groups, but is especially persuasive with older generations, who have lived through the years when medical breakthroughs in the treatment of illness has appeared to be most striking. Older people are aware of their increased susceptibility to illness, are generally too grateful for medical care, accepting without question the value of what they receive. Indeed, more than any other generation, they are made aware of their dependence upon medical assistance, and they have increasingly handed over personal responsibility for their health, accepting too willingly their dependence on medical help, harbouring instead a debilitating pessimism about the nature of old age.

Allopathy does have a useful, but spurious and misguided social advantage in this respect, for it allows individuals to believe that illness is not their fault, and that both the prevention and remedy for disease is not our responsibility. Diseases are seen as discrete entities invading our bodies. The 'germ invasion theory' has suited the human ego, which does not wish to face the realities of life. Most people prefer to believe that illness is the result of external forces, striking randomly through misfortune or bad luck, rather than as a consequence of personal lifestyle, social stress, or environmental pollution. The individual merely 'catches them'; locating the biological cause, and getting rid of it, becomes the responsibility of medicine. It is easier for people to believe that disease is external to normal life, not part of it, and that someone else should assume responsibility for making us better.

Medicalization and ageism form a dynamic and effective partnership. The ageing process is widely accepted as an explanation for illness and decline, with the fear of ageing representing a powerful component in the medicalization of old age. And the medical assumption that the main, perhaps the sole, determinant of health, is biological, is a powerful factor in ageism.

Implicit in medical propaganda are claims that older people live longer because of medical success, indeed, that they owe their continuing existence to medical science. Whilst the claim is suspect, it is widely accepted. Certainly, the idea that illness should be corrected by the medical profession is naive for two reasons.

First, allopathic medicine has few answers to the chronic health problems of old age. Older people are often told that 'nothing can be done', that their ailments are the inevitable consequence of ageing. Medical success with former 'killer' diseases has not been matched by the performance with the chronic, wasting diseases associated with old age. There is no cure for rheumatism, arthritis, chronic bronchitis, emphysema, chronic digestive problems, and for degenerative illnesses, such as multiple sclerosis and motor neurone disease, and there is no cure for mental illness in all its guises.

The tendency to blame such conditions on old age leaves the amelioration of these conditions, by relieving pain, discomfort and immobility, an acceptable alternative to curing them. Yet whilst drugs can sometimes bring about dramatic alleviation of symptoms, the solutions offered can be at best ineffective, and at worst give rise to further complications.

The second problem, discussed in more detail in Chapter 4, is that doctors usually take little account of the social and emotional setting in which many older people live. The sickest older people tend to be those who live lonely, isolated lives, a product of low income, lack of social role, and low morale, all of which can lead to anger, depression and sickness. Medical treatment using antidepressants and tranquillizers clearly misses the real needs of such people.

Yet the problem is deeper. The failure of medicine to produce effective treatment has led to practise with ageing people being considered an inferior, neglected, second-rate medical priority. This arises from ageist assumptions that consider old age to be a 'natural' process, for which there is no medical solution, just a lingering process of decline, ending in death. By implication, there is nothing heroic, interesting, or challenging in this ageist perception; the process of growing old is seen as merely a warehousing task, representing an unacceptable medical failure for a profession devoted to saving life through miracle cures, and heroic intervention.

Yet the medical neglect of older people does not more than mirror the priorities of other professional groups. Older people have long been considered the 'Cinderella' group of the social work profession. This is doubly debilitating, depressing not only professional work with older people, but confirming the low expectations many older people have about ageing, health, and their personal control over the future.

THE SOCIAL ROLE OF MEDICINE

From fetus to the grave, everyone is now subject to life-long medical supervision. Medical decisions have the power to encroach on the freedom of individuals, purely on the basis of assessments of their medical condition.

The social power of medicine is based on the operation of the sick role, a concept elaborated by Parsons (1970). The sick role determines appropriate behaviour for sick individuals. People adjudged to be sick are not held responsible for their incapacity, and are exempted from their usual social obligations. However, in return, it is expected that sick people should make every effort to become well again, and so are expected to comply with the conditions laid down by medical professionals. Failure to do so removes the individual from the sick role, labels them as 'philanderers', and stops entitlement to the social benefits of being sick.

The sick role is the basis of medical power. Making people 'legitimately' sick is as implicit in the power of doctors as their ability to make them better. The medical profession judges who is sick, who is well; who is fit, who is unfit; what is to be done to those who are sick; and, ultimately, to determine who is and who is not entitled to welfare benefits. Legal sanctions can be applied if there is any abuse of the system. Medical decisions also have an impact on many other, non-medical matters, deciding who can drive a car, who may be incarcerated in prisons or mental institutions, and who can take part in certain occupations. They even have to confirm that dead people are, in fact, dead.

Medicine is used to confirm older people in their unemployed social role outside of the labour market, their low social status, and low expectations. When younger people become sick, they are entitled to the benefits, and subject to the expectations of the sick role. Similarly, medicine helps to shape the social role of older people, who are unable to work by virtue of their age, and so are technically considered to be 'sick'. But unlike other groups, there is less pressure to overcome this form of ageist sickness and disability. Older people are expected to be ill simply on the basis of their chronological age. Nor does their 'sickness' cause loss of income, a threat to their employment status, or any other major social consequence. This not only makes the experience of 'sickness' different, but also makes recovery a lower medical priority.

Indeed, some older people, who want to be cared for and looked after, or who are feeling sorry for themselves, or seek increased attention, make use of this, and allow themselves to be confirmed inappropriately into the sick role.

There is a considerable amount of medication prescribed for reasons other than purely medical ones. The social control of 'deviant' individuals, whose behaviour for whatever reason is considered difficult, is often accomplished through medication and, in some cases, through surgical procedures. Medication is a quick, readily available, and relatively cheap method for dealing with such problems and difficulties. Such medical techniques are widely practised with 'difficult' older people. In the absence of better solutions, or the absence of time or priority to find them, medication is used to quieten difficult people, to combat wandering, and to sedate those who regularly complain. It is also used with people who suffer pain for which there is no other relief. This is often used to salve the conscience, and make life easier for carers, rather than for any real benefit to the individual concerned, for:

... such behaviour, labelled often as difficult, or even deviant, is rarely random or meaningless. The person is trying to communicate with his environment, trying to get across a scream for help. Unfortunately, the common answer is that the environment considers and treats the symptom as a disease, instead of listening to the message and seeking the real cause.

(Gidley and Shears, 1988)

Medication prevents the development of other techniques. The benzodiazepines can again be used to demonstrate this. These drugs make it more difficult for the individual to learn alternative strategies for coping with the stresses of life. The same effect can perhaps be obtained by other means, through music, art, physical exercise, a satisfying job, a loving relationship, and a host of other human activities all provide their own rewards and tranquillity. (Scrutton, 1989).

This analysis would appear to suggest that a wider, more balanced, more realistic view of health should be developed. Allopathic medicine alone cannot deliver better health. It can cure a number of conditions, and can relieve the symptoms in many others. It can help in managing long-term, chronic illness. It can save lives, although perhaps fewer than usually accepted. It can sometimes prolong life, even when it is not able to overcome illness. What medicine cannot do is to alter susceptibility to illness. It does not improve resistance to infection, or reduce the chances of contracting disease. It is singularly unsuccessful in stopping the recurrence of many chronic conditions suffered by many older people. For this, older people have to look elsewhere.

4

An holistic approach: the causes of illness in old age

Health is a vital component in the quality of life of older people. The definition of good health has, in recent times, been subject to a process of reduction, now indicating little more than the absence of illness and disease. Good health, however, is clearly much more than this, as the World Health Organization recognized when it defined it as 'a complete physical, mental and social well-being and not merely the absence of disease or infirmity'.

Older people, more than any other group, have cause to question dominant medical practice, yet they rarely do so. In order to widen the parameters of health, many questions need to be asked about the real contribution of allopathic medicine to the health of older people.

- Does allopathic medicine provide older people with superior health care?
- Is medical expertise always necessary for those who are unwell?
- Is allopathic medical intervention always beneficial to the recipient?
- Is allopathic medicine justified in taking credit for older people living longer?
- What can older people do for themselves in maintaining good health?
- Are there alternative forms of medicine which can play a role in the health care of older people?

Yet the first question has to concern the causes of illness in old age and, in particular, to challenge the idea that it is always, or mostly, concerned with age. There have been older people throughout history who have demonstrated that it is possible to age without illness, to maintain health, mobility and lucidity of mind, long into old age. Older people can live without significant illness or pain, whilst still accepting the inevitable consequences of the ageing process. There are many examples of famous individuals continuing to live, work, and lead a normal life into advanced old age. Picasso was still painting at 91, Toscanini still conducting at 89, and the example of many others, such as Somerset Maugham, Bertrand Russell, and Michael Tippett, suggests that there are answers to healthy ageing which are concerned with factors other than medical support. In his examination of longevity, Georgakas (1980) came to this conclusion:

> After so much human effort has been expended to find some exotic 'secret' to long life, it is somewhat ironic that the simplest life-styles and some of the most natural bodily responses are key longevity factors. Rather than extending the life-span or rejuvenating the body, prolongevous habits maintain the body's resistance to premature ageing.

The re-emergence of personal control is a major theme of this book. It is important that the role of medicine is placed where it belongs: to advise, to utilize knowledge and skill where appropriate, and to treat *in extremis*. But, ultimately, the central role must be played by the individual. Health is concerned with factors that remain within personal control, with each individual in control to a degree few would recognize.

This control is possible, regardless of age, whenever ageing is seen as a time of potential growth. However, this will not be possible unless the quality of life enjoyed by older people can be extended. Thus, it is important to concentrate upon an important distinction: not on the extension of life, but an extension of the quality of life.

There is a difficult paradox in this view. On the one hand, the individual needs to come to terms with the natural process of decline and death, whilst at the same time emphasizing the importance of not passively accepting, or giving in to it at any particular age. The paradox results from two different aspects of reality. The first concerns the mortality of human life. This cannot, and certainly should not, be denied, but accepted as part of the life process, as it is in Oriental traditions. The second is that the major contributory factors which lead to decline and death are not influenced by natural biological forces or, indeed, by medical ability to divert them, but are concerned with life-factors over which the individual has considerable control.

The problem with old age is not reaching it, but arriving in a condition that makes it a pleasure rather than a misery. This raises the question of whether it is possible, by taking better care of our body, to prevent illness becoming a major problem in old age. Fulder (1983) was doubtful, stating that:

> ... our medical system is designed to get you to old age but is not concerned with the state in which you arrive there.

The premise of the germ theory, developed by Pasteur, Koch and Lister, tends to suggest that disease has a single physiological cause. The most important development of recent years has been to recognize that the causes of disease are multiple, and that the impact of personal, social and environmental factors are equally, if not more, significant.

> All natural phenomena are the result of complex inter-relationships; all manifestations of human disease are the consequence of the interplay of body, mind and environment. This situation creates a difficult dilemma for physicians and medical scientists. They recognize that the analytic breakdown of the problems of disease into their component parts never results in a true picture; yet they know from practical experience that the artificial reduction of these problems into the consti-tuent parts, or their conversion into simpler models, is an absolute necessity for scientific progress.
>
> (Dubos, 1970)

This has restricted the development of a holistic viewpoint from within allopathic medicine. The powerful impact on health of social and environmental factors continues to be largely ignored. The air we breathe undeniably induces disease and disabilty; stress violates our social life; our diet is contaminated; but medicine does not deal with any of these factors, except at the level of symptoms.

A broader perspective is necessary in which declining health is seen to arise at six levels. It is our understanding or, perhaps, misunderstanding of the relative importance of these different levels that has had a major impact on current views of health in old age.

1. NATURAL MORBIDITY

Whilst it remains too easy to dismiss illness as an inevitable conse-quence of ageing, it has to be recognized that gradual decline and eventual death are important factors in the health of older people. The most fundamental aspect of death and decline arises from the natural and irresistible process of ageing. Life is not forever; nothing which lives can escape its own mortality. Decline and death is ultimately a natural and inevitable process. Indeed, older people are often more aware than most of this universal fact of all life.

Normal ageing tends to have significant effects on health. The skin becomes thinner; height decreases; muscle strength declines; blood vessels harden; the lungs lose elasticity; the gums shrink leading to tooth loss; kidney and liver function declines; reflexes become slower; the brain loses weight; and the sense of taste, sight and hearing diminish. Whilst such changes might be considered normal ageing processes, their speed and severity varies so much between individuals that it is clear that they are not entirely inevitable; there are other factors that determine their speed and extent.

The problem is that 'natural' ageing processes are too readily transformed into an unwarranted pessimism about the ageing process, and the quality of life that is possible. The 'inevitability' of decline is too often used to explain physical ailments which are more accurately associated with disease.

Whilst medicine should not have an impact on the natural process of death and decline, there is implicit within medical ideology the suggestion that death is something that should be overcome, perhaps most clearly seen in the development and use of life-support systems, whose use is often continued long after hopes for survival, with an acceptable quality of life, is gone. Organ transplantation, undertaken in the name of 'health', owes more to the non-acceptance of death than a commitment to life. In these and other ways, medicine makes promises it cannot deliver. More crucially, it undermines social acceptance of an inevitable and integral process of ageing.

2. ILLNESS AND DISEASE

Whilst ageing witnesses an increasing susceptibility to disease, illness can occur at any time and does not signify that the patient is ageing. It is the primary focus of medicine to help recovery from ill health. Medical practice is increasingly reluctant to accept that illness is inevitable, and is prepared to go to considerable lengths to treat the illnesses of younger people. Older people do not always get such a good deal, so it is important to emphasize that ageing is not a disease, and that there is a vital distinction between natural decline and illness.

> To be old is not to be ill; and to be ill and old is
> as treatable as being young and ill.

Medicine fails older people in its tendency to concentrate on acute disease, and its lack of success treating the chronic degenerative diseases that afflict so many ageing people. Medicine tends to be curative rather than preventative. Doctors can diagnose arthritis, but cannot predict its development. Medical diagnosis, as Fulder (1983) states, is often too much, too late. Medicine claims to have extended life expectation, yet its failure in this respect has not enhanced the quality of life experience. Indeed, by extending life whilst failing to reduce pain and debility, medicine has made ageing more, rather than less, fearful.

Nor is the failure confined to prognosis. Everyone can contract disease, but the circumstances in which some people become sick while others, similarly situated, do not, are not adequately explained by allopathic medicine. Exposure to a pathogen may be a necessary condition, but it is not a sufficient one. Viral exposure results in disease only when the exposed individual is in a 'receptive' state.

This receptivity is affected by a variety of other factors. Heredity is probably the most important factor which determines health and longevity. Whilst individuals cannot change this, it is possible to alter many factors in order to give our inherited constitution a better chance. To illustrate this Gore (1973) used a horticultural parallel. If a plant, bred from good stock, is allowed to grow, but then deprived of water, it will wilt and die, no matter how splendid its inherited constitution, because its environment is no longer able to support life.

There are doubts about medical claims to have extended life expectancy. The contrary view is that it has increased through improved diet, public health improvements, and a variety of anti-poverty measures rather than any significant improvement in medical intervention. Statistics concerning life expectation are misleading. Improved longevity can be indicated by more people surviving childbirth and infancy than any direct benefit to older people. Life expectancy for those reaching maturity is little higher now than 100 years ago.

3. LIFESTYLE FACTORS

The relationship between lifestyle and good health has been recognized for many centuries. Hippocrates, over 2000 years ago, advocated fresh air, exercise and good food, sound advice which has been repeated throughout history. Only in more recent times, blinded by the apparent miracles of medical science, have these simple truths has been overtaken in importance by medical intervention.

Many conditions associated with ageing have their roots in personal lifestyle. They include habits such as smoking, drugs, excessive drinking, inadequate nutrition and exercise. There are also personal factors, such as divorce, boredom and frustration, all known to affect health. If their action is slow and imperceptible, they operate with such certainty that it is these factors, rather than our genes or the invasion of bacteria and viruses, that determine health expectations.

Two major consequences arise from recognizing the importance of lifestyle, one favourable, the other unfavourable to older people. The problem is that lifestyle factors can lead to explanations for ill health based on 'personal pathology', the result of personal foolishness or inadequacy. This is the 'victim-blaming' approach to health care. Just as illness can be dismissed as the result of ageing, it is also easy to dismiss disease as the result of ill-considered, personal lifestyle. This often results in many older people refusing to see their doctor because they find too often that either their age, or their foolishness, is blamed for their ailments.

Personal pathology as an explanation for the condition of weaker social groups, of whom older people are just one example, is totally inadequate. Such explanations intimate that people with more money, power or influence, have obtained their position because of some mental or physical superiority. Those with a vested interest in the maintenance of the social status quo support these arguments with a number of self-justifying scientific theories, of which Social Darwinism is one, explaining social inequity as a process of natural selection, with rewards accruing to the worthy, and misfortune being singled out for the less worthy.

Yet to ignore lifestyle factors for this reason is not sensible. Much illness is the result of life habits practised over many years. This indicates, helpfully, that the solution rests as much in prevention through personal decisions than cures contained in a bottle of tranquillizers. Lifestyle factors should not be used to 'blame' the individual, but to emphasize the importance of personal rather than medical decisions in the maintenance of health. Maintaining health is a conscious process, not a game of chance against unknown odds, or against diseases which strike at random. Personal commitment is required in order to remain healthier, for longer. The relationship between health and personal choice is not exclusive; there are many other factors, but it is important to realize that the maintenance of health involves a significant degree of personal choice.

Lifestyle factors stress the importance of self-care in maintaining health. The elements that constitute a 'healthy' lifestyle, and the habits, activities and attitudes which can produce ill health are now well known. They include emotional factors, such as unresolved anger, shock or grief, and unrequited or unexpressed passions; there is low self-esteem, and a failure to think of personal needs; a lack of purpose in life, especially in the social sphere; a lack of physical exercise; and nutritional imbalances that deprive the body of essential requirements. Allied to all these factors are certain habits which often arise from them, particularly smoking and drinking.

All these factors can have particular significance to older people, although too often they are presumed to lay outside the health care agenda. Conventional medicine places less emphasis on preventative methods of health maintenance, and more on complex and complicated cures, mostly directed at acute disease. In developing these, the importance of lifestyle factors have been significantly discounted.

The implication seems to be that individuals can live riotously, abuse themselves, and then have a replacement heart; but the answer to ill health in old age should not be medication or surgery. Drugs, bypass surgery, or a new heart should not be considered an alternative to changing the habits which cause heart disease. A wider approach to health should address the causes, not just the symptoms, concentrating on individual decisions about lifestyle which are under direct, personal control.

Lifestyle decisions are bound to the dominant ideology of the time. Older generations live in ways inextricably connected with the habits, tastes, fashions and fads that existed during their childhood and youth. Many are now known to be unhealthy, for example, smoking was considered to be sophisticated, and the consumption of alcohol, in moderation, quite harmless, when our older generations were younger.

Health in old age is, in part, a legacy of past lifestyle. The human body possesses remarkable powers of adaptation and tolerance. It can cope with various abuses from which it does not suffer at the time, or from which it soon recovers. It is only with ageing that the main penalties are exacted, and the apparent tolerance of the body to abuse ceases. Many degenerative diseases can be seen as the ultimate price the body has to pay for past misdemeanours.

This gives rise to the idea that it is 'too late' to avoid the damage already done in the past. This is not so. If health has been damaged, it does not necessitate continuation, either from the ageist idea that it is 'too late', or the ostrich-like attitude that 'it has not hurt us up to now ... '. The individual can modify long-standing life habits, and there is evidence to suggest that changes in lifestyle can affect health even in later old age (Fulder (1983); Walford (1983)).

Many health decisions are a matter for national education, as much as individual choice. Death from heart disease in the UK is now amongst the highest in world. Previously, this unwanted record was held by the USA, Finland, Australia and New Zealand, but deaths there have been dramatically reduced primarily through an education programme that supported the conscious adoption of simple lifestyle changes, more powerful in their health impact than anything that could be achieved by medical intervention.

It is useful to illustrate some aspects of lifestyle which are now known to be detrimental to health in later years.

Alcohol and drug abuse

The drinking of alcohol is socially accepted, legally sanctioned, and its ready availability obscures its powerful drug affect. Its popularity rests upon its apparent ability to aid sociability, arising from its impact in dulling the higher centres of the brain, reducing self-consciousness and worry, and apparently soothing anxiety and relieving tension. The popular perception, often confirmed by doctors, is that an occasional drink is not detrimental to health, and that alcohol is actually good for health.

Although drinking tends to decline with age, older drinkers are more likely to drink alone, at home, in an attempt to escape their depressed social role (Eckardt, 1978). Even alcoholism in old age is more common than generally realized, so it is important that the dangers of alcohol are more widely understood. In old age, moderate consumption of alcohol on a regular basis can have harmful consequences, complicating many disease processes.

The cumulative effects of even relatively small quantities of alcohol makes great demands upon the liver and kidneys. Older people, particularly women who can cope with significantly less alcohol at any age, are particularly vulnerable to ill health through alcohol consumption because of their reduced kidney and liver function. Alcohol is a toxic and addictive drug, which acts on the nervous system and brain, initially as a stimulant, but eventually with depressant effects. Alcohol is absorbed through the small intestine, detoxified by enzymes in the liver and, in the process, liver cells are destroyed. During heavy drinking, this enzyme cannot cope, and alcohol is allowed into the bloodstream. With regular drinking, the liver is unable to repair itself, leading eventually to cirrhosis, which disables and kills large numbers of older people.

Long-term excessive consumption of alcohol has been associated with blood disorders such as anaemia, lung disease, heart muscle damage, increased susceptibility to infection, digestive ulcers, pancreatitis (a fatal disease of the pancreas), neuropathy (a progressive and debilitating disease of the nervous system), and cancer of the mouth, throat and oesophagus. Over a long period, it can lead to cirrhosis, the fatal inflammation of the liver.

Large quantities of alcohol can lead to the degeneration of the central nervous system, and damage the nerve cells in the brain, affecting memory and concentration. Alcohol acts by depressing the nervous system, and taken in excess it impairs intellectual functioning, causing stupor, unconsciousness and, eventually, coma and death. The symptoms of alcohol abuse are often difficult to distinguish from forms of mental infirmity, poor memory, incontinence, depression and shakiness, and it is perhaps a salutary understanding that the brains of relatively young alcoholics have been found in post-mortem to be similar in appearance to those of much older non-alcoholics. It is suggested that the chronic use of alcohol may 'speed up' the normal ageing process of the brain, and can produce premature ageing. It is known that alcohol's effects on memory range from 'cocktail-party deficits' to almost total memory loss for recent events (Eckardt, 1978).

Prolonged drinking can also harm the absorbtion of certain foods, leading to malnutrition and vitamin deficiency, particularly folic acid and vitamin B. In addition, it has been argued that alcohol can lead to premature hair loss, and ageing of the skin. It can alter the therapeutic effect of drugs, such as pain killers, anticoagulants, antibiotics, anticonvulsants, antihistamines, antihypertensives, diuretics, major tranquillizers, antidepressants, sedative-hypnotics, and even stimulants.

Smoking

Smoking is another socially accepted killer habit, increasing the risk of most serious diseases. Nicotine and carbon monoxide is inhaled into the lungs, from where it is absorbed into the bloodstream, and so passed directly to the heart and the rest of the body. Smoking is therefore implicated in most diseases, but most specifically for causing lung cancer, bronchitis, emphysema and heart disease.

Nicotine is an addictive drug which increases adrenaline in the bloodstream, raising pulse rate, and increasing blood-pressure; it aids the build-up of cholesterol, furs up the coronary arteries, and thereby reduces the amount of blood reaching the heart. At the same time, carbon monoxide reduces the oxygen-carrying haemoglobin in the blood supply to the heart muscle, increasing the heart's oxygen requirement. This leads ultimately to arteriosclerosis, heart disease and stroke.

Smoking introduces toxic substances directly to the lungs, irritating the lining of bronchi, and leading to inflammation and secretion of mucous in lung tissue. This eventually reduces its ability to absorb oxygen, leading initially to breathlessness, and eventually to bronchitis, emphysema and cancer of the mouth, throat and lungs.

Many older people counter antismoking arguments by claiming that their survival indicates that it has done them little harm. Yet survival has been achieved despite tobacco, not because of it. Most smokers die earlier than they would otherwise have done, but those who have died are no longer around to attest to its dangers. It is known that the harmful effects of smoking, if compensated for by good diet, can be less severe; smoking in Spain has been found to be less harmful because the staple diet includes more fruit and vegetables, and less animal fat. Yet smoking also harms appetite and diet, making this safety feature less achievable.

It would appear that it is never too late to give up. The risk of death or disease has been found to decline the moment the habit stops. The argument that, 'I've been smoking for so long now that it isn't going to make any real difference' is simply an excuse to carry on the habit (Ashton and Davies, 1986).

Smoking is perhaps too closely identified with death, and not sufficiently with the pain and suffering that accompany the illnesses it produces, particularly in later years. Younger smokers are more susceptible to death than their older counterparts, presumably as those individuals who are particularly susceptible to smoking are eliminated from the population at an earlier stage, and those who survive are more robust, or luckier colleagues (Ashton and Davies, 1986). The real cost of smoking should be expressed in terms of ill health and quality of life rather than premature death. The irony of the 'you can only die once' argument, based on the ageist attitude that people do not wish to live into depressing old age, is that smoking may not kill them, but instead ensure that they endure the very suffering and disability in old age that they fear.

Smoking is a conscious and deliberate pollution of our body. The dangers of smoking are now well understood, and commonly accepted, even by smokers, so the survival of the habit needs to be reassessed. Each smoker has powerful reasons for continuing to overcome the rationale and logic of self-interest. The underlying compulsion is an addiction to nicotine, which many smokers cannot acknowledge, or are unable to act upon, for such an admission underlines personal weakness.

For non-smokers, the dangers of passive smoking has to be considered. The Independent Scientific Committee on Smoking and Health recently reported that non-smokers are between 10% and 30% more likely to contract lung cancer if consistently exposed to tobacco smoke, pointing out that the smoke from cigarette ends contains greater concentrations of toxic chemicals than the smoke filtered into smoker's lungs.

4. THE SOCIAL WORLD

Our health is as intimately linked now with current social conditions as it was two centuries ago. Many improvements in health have been the direct result of improved housing, working conditions, diet, water supply, sewerage and garbage disposal. The link between social organization and health is hotly disputed. It has been claimed that capitalism and the class structure make people ill (Thunhurst, 1981; Mitchell, 1984; Doyle, 1983), but arguments suggesting that weaker social groups are disadvantaged by subtle forms of social injustice are usually castigated as being unscientific and emotive. Yet the logic of capitalism is that it does not matter if junk food, cigarettes, alcohol or other merchandise damage health, as long as it sells; that it does not matter if workers, or people living near factories are damaged so long as the product is made and sold. Whilst this is not a popular concept, many features of the social world are increasingly recognized as being fundamentally unhealthy.

The social world incorporates many emotional, social, political, and economic factors which all impinge upon health. Social organization provides different groups with different health experiences. There are diverse experiences of employment, housing, education, lifestyle, income-related nutritional experiences, and family circumstances. The particular health needs of women, and ethnic minority communities, have also to be considered within each of these, as do the needs of older people, as a 'marginalized', or under-privileged group.

The *Black Report* looked at these differences as they affected mortality and morbidity rates between social class groups (Whitehead *et al.*, 1988). It concluded that lower occupational groups had poorer health experiences at all stages of life, and that despite more than 30 years of an NHS committed to equalizing health care, there remained a marked class differential in standards of health care. The report argued that this arose from factors such as income, work experience, the work environment, unemployment, education, housing, transport, and the quality of diet. Each significantly affected health regardless of whether the illness was an everyday problem, such as back pain, a life-threatening illness, such as cancer or heart disease, or a chronic disabling disease, such as arthritis.

The Health Divide confirmed the findings of the *Black Report*, adding that occupational class differences applied equally to those aged over 65 (Whitehead *et al.*, 1988). Whilst sickness eventually occurred regardless of class, lower occupational groups experienced it earlier. The report concluded that this was a major source of social inequality. Both reports argued that behaviour relevant to the maintenance of health is located within social structures, associated with, and reinforced by, class, the division of labour, and the social distribution of rewards. These factors structure the distinctive class responses towards lifestyle and living habits.

Both reports left little doubt that social and financial hardship is paid for in terms of human health, and that those who suffer most were likely to experience greater ill health in old age. The structural argument which underlay both reports is that poorer people become ill more often because they have greater exposure to health-damaging factors over which they have little control. Factory and mine workers experience hazardous working conditions, the fear of redundancy, and the pressures of productivity agreements related to pay. Associations have been made between unemployment and health with increased incidence of depression, suicide, cirrhosis of the liver, and raised blood-pressure. Damp housing has been linked to bronchitis, asthma, and other respiratory diseases associated with old age, and the financial problems of maintaining a warm, dry home. Low income means constant worry about paying for food, rent, and the prospect of hunger and eviction. Retired people on basic pensions die of hypothermia because they cannot buy sufficient fuel, not because they are growing old. How such factors related to the experience of older people was outlined in the *Black Report*:

In old age the relationship between income and the capacity to protect personal health is stronger perhaps than at any other time in the life cycle, and in general it is likely that individuals who are well endowed through generous index-linked pension schemes will lead the healthiest, the most comfortable and the longest lives after retirement. These material fortunes or misfortunes of old age are closely linked with occupational class during the working life. To have secure employment and an above-average income when one is at work is to be better able to provide for one's retirement. It is in this way that continuity in the distribution of material welfare is sustained, and inequalities in health perpetuated, from the cradle to the grave.

(Whitehead *et al.*, 1988)

Both reports recommended significant improvements in the material conditions of disadvantaged groups. Yet to respond to their radical conclusions would have considerable social and political implications. It would have a fundamental impact on the treatment of older people in respect of health-related factors, such as financial security, housing, and social role. As a basis for health care provision, it would involve a considerable social revolution. Opposition to the findings, particularly from those with a vested interest in social inequality, was not surprising.

The Establishment view prefers cultural and behavioral explanations, in which differential class patterns of ill health can be explained by reckless lifestyle choices. Ill health results from factors under personal control, that people ignore the advice of doctors, disregarding their future health. They have insufficient will-power and self-control to resist health-damaging practices, and but for their irresponsible behaviour, they would be healthier.

The suppression of the *Black Report*, with only 260 duplicated copies being made available, and the controversy over *The Health Divide*, which led to the disbanding of the Health Education Council, clearly illustrated that the Establishment places little emphasis on the impact that the social world has on health (Whitehead *et al.*, 1988). Our medical system continues to ignore the relationship between illness and the social forces destructive to it. The emphasis it places on the biological causation of disease suggests that whilst our minds might be affected by the social world, our bodies are only affected by the physical world through harmful pathogens, such as bacteria, viruses, alcohol, food, and carcinogens.

The social pressures which drive people to smoke, drink and eat badly are ignored. People persist in health-destructive behaviour when they have little hope, and this can be particularly important for older people. Considerable psychological stress accompanies forced retirement, boredom at home, financial uncertainty, fears about ill health, loss of loved ones, isolation, the lack of alternative sources of enjoyment. Older people often cannot see value in self-denial in order to invest in a future in which they do not believe, making this area of understanding particularly important for the health of older people.

Improving health at this level is less the province of medicine than politics. The problem is not inadequate knowledge, but the social and political will to ensure that everyone enjoys a standard of health that arises from a decent income, and good working and living conditions, all of which can enable older people to feel in control of their lives.

The germ theory of disease has an enormous impact on medical science, but germs require the right environment in which to grow. The social conditions in which many older people live are ideal seedbeds for bacteria and viruses to thrive.

5. EMOTIONAL ASPECTS OF HEALTH

The influence of emotional life on health has been known at least since the second century BC, when Greek physicians attributed cancer to a 'melancholy disposition'. Contemporary evidence is now confirming significant links between cancer and stress. Unfortunately, the theories of Descartes, that the mind and body were divisible, erected a formidable barrier that persists in Western medicine today.

Medicine demands scientific and logical explanations, and refuses any idea, however old and well-tested, that emotions are connected with health care. The difficulty of proving scientific links between emotion and physical health means that allopathic medicine tends to neglect emotional aspects of health, concentrating instead on the association between depression and chemical imbalances in the body. Its reliance on drugs fails to recognize that chemical imbalances themselves are probably the result of emotional and social factors, thus to respond with tranquillizers, or antidepressant medication may deal with the symptoms, but fails to address the causation.

Despite this, there is a gradual reassessment of the links between the mind and physical illness. Eastern medical practice has always believed that illness originates from an imbalance between the mind and body. Psychoanalysis has sharpened Western medical awareness of the interplay between mental and bodily functioning, leading to the recognition that many kinds of stimuli can affect both psychic and organic processes. Psychosomatic medicine, concerned with the causation of organic disease by mental disturbances, is gradually recognizing that physical conditions can be induced by unresolved emotional problems or conflicts. The attitude which dismissed 'psychosomatic' illness as a euphemism for illness that did not exist, as there was no identifiable physical cause, is now slowly declining.

Such acceptance could revolutionize our approach to disease. Ornstein and Sobel (1988) argued that it is pointless to throw money into medicine, which continues to separate mind and body, and that the key to future health is to recognize the power of the mind on health. If illness is caused in minds, the remedy for that illness should be sought there. Pelletier (1978) also argues for a holistic approach to preventing illness caused by stress.

Disease is the outcome of a multitude of life experiences, accumulated tensions, anxieties and stresses, and the habits adopted to cope with them. These accumulate throughout life, eventually affecting health in old age. Stress is increasingly used to explain emotional factors in illness. The human body is capable of dealing with a degree of stress; this ability is necessary for good health. However, excessive stress over long periods has been linked with such ailments as headaches, stiffness, aches and pains, tiredness and lack of energy, sleeplessness, nervousness, violent emotional outburts, and an increasing dependence upon palliatives, such as smoking, alcohol, over-eating and drugs. Chronic stress has been associated with susceptibility to infections, such as influenza and pneumonia, the development of ulcers, cancer, and is considered an important contributor to mental illness.

The process can be explained physiologically. Stress causes muscles to contract, using oxygen at an accelerated rate. Oxygen provides muscles with energy, but contraction through stress deprives them of oxygen by narrowing the blood vessels that transport oxygen-laden blood. The muscles are forced to feed on limited reserves, depleting the oxygen supply so that muscles are unable to function properly, eventually deteriorating. Similarly, stress can damage the heart and blood vessels, raising blood-pressure and cholesterol levels. The stressed brain can also become incapable of co-ordinating the complex movements required for daily routines, thereby increasing the frequency of accidents.

Stress is an increasingly important modern symptom, associated with social pressures which impose a variety of duties and obligations on the individual. Older people are subjected to anxiety and stress, despite the patronisingly ageist idea that they live carefree and restful lives in contented retirement. Stress results from an inability to achieve personal objectives, and many older people are confronted with competitive, aggressive, and stressful patterns of social life, which subtly produce anger, fears and apprehension, which remain debilitating obstacles to leading a healthy life.

Older people also face emotional stress connected with ageism. The psychology of ageism remains largely unexplored, but centres on the fears and depressed expectations of growing old. Medical ageism can be particularly depressing, with the self-congratulatory rhetoric taking credit for extending life expectation on the one hand, and the passive and practical support of ageist paradigms of health on the other. This needs to be challenged not only in respect of its accuracy, but on its impact on self-image. Older people need support if they are to escape attitudes that can be damaging to health. The struggle for survival in the modern world is not fought exclusively against the invasion of microbes, but with our nerves, feelings, and emotions.

Since stress is largely unavoidable, the aim should be to minimize its harmful effects by finding healthier outlets for nervous energies. *It is the way individuals deal with stress, as much as stress itself that determines its impact on health.* With older people, stress often leads to apathy and depression, to exhaustion, and the breakdown of physical health. Stress is better dealt with by more, not less, activity and excitement. It is important to increase the time spent on exercise and recreational pursuits, and in relaxation through music, art, or even yoga, hypnotherapy, biofeedback and Alexander technique, which are all important, but neglected, treatments for stress-related illness.

6. ENVIRONMENTAL FACTORS

In order to analyse the effects of environmental factors on health and on disease, it is ... necessary to keep in mind that man's life always involves a complex interplay between the conditions of the present and the attributes he has retained from his evolutionary and experiential past.

(Dubos, 1970)

The contribution of environmental factors to human ill health remains controversial, its full impact still denied by those responsible for economic, industrial and technological growth, and the resulting pollution. Scientific evidence is not always entirely objective. Even the highest statistical probability linking environmental factors and health is not sufficient if they do not correspond to dominant ideas, or are seen to be detrimental to the interests of powerful social interests. It has taken many decades to prove the point against tobacco; it will probably take many more to substantiate the case against environmental pollution.

The integrity of the 'science' which permits this has to be questioned. The demand for proof beyond all reasonable doubt disqualifies connections between the environment and illness, indicating the value to the Establishment of scientific method; medical science often insists that without 'proof' nothing can, or indeed, needs to be done. The difficulty of proving direct relationships between a single environmental cause, and a single health effect in a world with so many variables, denies a wider understanding of the causation of disease, and leaves allopathic medicine able to function without reference to the environment in which the individual lives.

This century has witnessed unprecedented environmental change. Air, water and soil, the essences of all life, are becoming increasingly susceptible to pollution as the human population increases, and continues to treat the Earth without proper respect. Environmental pollution is now difficult to avoid, and a wider understanding of health must take account of the dangers of living in a polluted world. Concern usually centres on its impact on child health because of their lower tolerance levels, mainly involving statistics on birth defects, and the development of cancer. Yet the cumulative effects of pollution throughout adult life, allied with the reduced tolerance of older people, is rarely mentioned. Older people are exposed to a lifetime of work, with its frequent exposure to vibration, radiation, abnormal temperatures, noise, noxious chemicals and dangerous machinery, which must all take their toll.

There is a tendency, supported by science, to believe that the human body can adjust successfully to environmental pollution. Lists of 'tolerances' to chemical and other pollutants have been produced, showing that the human body can withstand pollution without damage to health, figures which are increasingly disputed, although not yet entirely discredited. Subtle propaganda which suggests that all life is dependent on chemicals, and that no chemical is entirely safe in all situations, should not obscure the difference between chemicals found in nature, and chemicals made in the laboratory; very few chemicals are carcinogenic, but most that are have been created artificially (Georgakas, 1980).

The human body does have considerable powers of adaptation. It has adapted to the carrot which contains carratatoxin, a potent nerve poison; to fish which contain small parts of arsenic; and to onions, olives, melons, potatoes and many other natural foods which contain similar harmful substances. But it is likely that adaptive powers have had insufficient time to accommodate the rapid industrialization of the last two centuries, with an ever-increasing quantity of toxic and allergenic chemicals being put into food, air and drinking water. Our adaptation to this assault is probably less satisfactory than is supposed.

Indeed, the most disturbing aspect of human adaptation is, paradoxically, that very adaptability, which allows it to adjust to conditions and habits that will eventually destroy the values most characteristic of human life. Biological adaptability has led to the passive acceptance of undesirable environmental conditions, to the extent that there is real danger that man will progressively forget the values that constitute the most precious and unique quality of human life (Dubos, 1970).

Scientific compromise is already subject to increasing doubt; the accumulation of sub-lethal doses, whilst not immediately harmful, may damage health in the longer term, thus making older people particularly vulnerable. Explanations for the vast health differences between individuals must involve looking beyond known risk factors, like drinking and smoking, to examine less easily quantifiable aspects of modern life.

Air pollution is rampant. Greater quantities of harmful substances are inhaled through the lungs than in any other way. Those people living in urban industrial areas experience considerable atmospheric pollution from vehicles and factories. In the early 1950s, a series of smogs in London led to the passing of the Clean Air Act 1956. Smog was caused by industry pouring smoke containing corrosive gases into the atmosphere. Periodically, droplets of water containing corrosive acids would descend, which would eat away stone buildings. As Mackarness (1980) asserted, the impact of these acids on the lungs was not difficult to imagine.

Modern society continues to pour toxic gases into the atmosphere. Our environment is becoming steadily more contaminated with synthetic derivatives of petroleum-derived hydrocarbons and other pollutants, which commonly induce disease in susceptible people – even in minute dosage. The cumulative effects of constant exposure to industrial dusts, containing sulphur dioxide and other pollutants, has contributed to the widespread development of emphysema, asthma and chronic bronchitis, and other respiratory diseases. Lead from vehicle petrol fumes can seriously affect the brain and central nervous systems of children, a problem that was scientifically denied for many years. Allergy to tobacco and petrol fumes is also implicated in bronchitis, although not as well recognized a cause as viral infection (Mackarness, 1976).

Yet people living in non-industrialized areas also suffer from pollution. Pesticides and herbicides are on sale for unrestricted use by farmers, horticulturists and gardeners. Initially developed as chemical weapons of war, they have been modified to control pests ranging from insects, weeds, mites, fungi, worms and vermin. This chemical destruction of pests on farms and gardens has become so commonplace that nobody now thinks of the potential dangers to human health. The complexity of agricultural sprays and chemicals is now so great, and their use so widespread, that overdoses can produce deformity and deficiency; and it is known that they can produce acute reactions in the central nervous system, and are suspected to contribute to many other modern ailments (Mackarness, 1980). The inhalation of minute doses of such chemicals can produce a variety of problems, including irritability, nausea, excitement followed by depression, weakness, sweating, contracted pupils, tears, runny nose, drooling from the mouth, loss of appetite, laboured breathing, slow heartbeat, tremor, muscular twitching, gastro-intestinal disturbance, involuntary urination and defecation and mental disturbance (Carlson, 1975; Watson, 1972). Many skin conditions are linked to contact with either household or industrial chemicals.

There are many other poisons in common domestic use that can induce psychochemical responses – Watson (1972) provides examples ranging from mothballs, to spraying with insect killer, to the fumes of drying paint. Many common household products offered as chemical remedies for household activities ranging from hair sprays, disinfectants, paint, floor wax, chlorine bleach, cleaning fluids and insecticides, all pollute the air.

The implicaiton for consumers of such chemicals are considerable. They have entered the food chain, our clothes, carpets and floorboards. Traces are found in rainfall, the water supply, and most commercially produced food. They are found within human fat tissue, in fetuses and mother's milk. Traces have been found even in Antarctic penguins.

Radiation is another problem, its links with illness being increasingly realized. The body can tolerate background atmospheric and

59

geological radiation, but denser pulses are known to cause premature ageing and cancer. Radiation is harmful because it produces free radicals, vicious reactive chemical fragments that reverberate through the body, causing widespread damage, interfering with the body's metabolism and cell reproduction. Cells damaged in this way can become cancerous. Radiation, for instance, remains the only known cause of leukaemia.

Electricity has become an essential feature of modern life, yet the effects of electrical appliances remains largely unknown. Microwave activity, produced in the generation and transmission of electricity, and brought into the home by an increasing plethora of electrical equipment, creates high-energy magnetic fields, and electro-magnetic radiation, which can affect human health by interacting with the body's own electrical field. High-tension power cables distort electromagnetic fields, and have been found to make people irritable and unwell, leading to headaches, drowsiness, congestion and even confusion. It might also contribute to hyperactivity, muscle weakness, and may even trigger multiple sclerosis (Mansfield, 1988).

One demonstration of the powerful impact of modern society is the way that many 'primitive' peoples have fallen prey to disease when they come into contact with Western civilization, which introduced infectious agents against which they had no resistance. Yet there is evidence that 'advanced' civilization is now suffering from the pollution it has created. Environmental factors now subject the body to a multiplicity of chemical and biological agents that are promoting disease. Whilst our immune system might ensure that most exposure does not immediately result in disease, as the body ages this adaptive response declines.

The importance of environmental factors can perhaps answer some of the more puzzling features of modern health. Why do so many people feel slightly 'under the weather'? Why do so many people suffer debilitating disorders, with obscure medical names? Myalgic encephalomyelitis (ME), or post-viral syndrome, attacks the central nervous system and muscles, causes pain, swelling, weakness and paralysis is one example. The 'sick-building syndrome' is another. Toxoplasmosis, or the 'yuppie flu', which incapacitated an athlete as fit as Sebastian Coe, is another. None are readily accepted as medical diseases, often being dismissed as psychiatric problems, or malingering.

What such complaints appear to have in common is the vague, non-specific nature of their symptoms, producing feelings of exhaustion, lethargy and general depression. Are they concerned with the stress of modern life, with environmental pollution, or the effect of both on the immune system? One suggestions is that the debilitating conditions may be allergic reactions to modern pollution. Tobacco, dust, pollens, spores, hair, textiles, animal dander and other particles can produce minor allergic reactions. Greater allergic effects result from foods, alcoholic drinks, drugs, odours, fumes and such chemical emanations as coal gas and petrol-engine hydrocarbons (Watson, 1972; Mackarness, 1976). Although the mechanisms and the exact consequences remain uncertain, the impact of pollution on all life forms certainly seems to be rebounding with increasing speed and vigour, not least on the species which produced it.

Cancer is now acknowledged to arise from environmental sources. Four out of five cancers are environmental in origin, caused by a range of toxic substances, called carcinogens. They are either inhaled, ingested or come into contact with the skin. Smoking, industrial chemicals and diet, including food additives, have all been implicated. Many argue that the role of industrial processes has been underplayed.

Environmental pollution affects everyone. The larger significance of pollution is that any alteration of natural conditions is likely to have unfavourable effects as all components of nature are interrelated and interdependent. Human life is not immune, but part of a highly integrated web. Acid rain will not just kill trees, lakes and rivers, and the fish who live in them; it will ultimately damage human health.

There may be little that an individual can do to avoid the health damage caused by environmental pollution. But it is possible for the individual to ventilate rooms, use natural furnishings, avoid tobacco smoke, extract kitchen fumes, and use lots of house plants. It is possible to be on guard against industrial pollutants, such as aerosols. It is possible to limit exposure to radiation by avoiding radiant and fan heaters, air-conditioners, fluorescent lighting, and televisions, and their effects can be reduced by the use of ionizers. A healthy diet can reject all adulterated food.

Reliance on medicine is less sensible, for it continues to focus on the cure of the human animal whose environment is destroying him (Carlson, 1975). Heart transplants are a ludicrously expensive way of dealing with heart disease caused by environmental factors, which have damaged not only the heart, but all blood vessels leading to it (Mackarness, 1980).

A WIDER PROBLEM, A WIDER APPROACH

Allopathic medicine sees disease as an organic, physical process, a malevolent intruder which has to be identified, fought and over-come. It fights invading pathogens, such as bacteria, viruses and toxins, which enter the body by chance, accident or misfortune. Each specific disease is believed to have its own cause, rooted in biochemical processes in which lifestyle, social relationships, emotions, and the environment play only a minor role. Even mental illness is assumed to be traceable to biochemical malfunctioning. The task of medicine is to identify the cause, and discover a cure, usually treating a particular part, or consisting of the straightforward suppression of symptoms. Any wider perspective has been essentially lost.

An holistic approach to health derives from the idea that the whole is greater than the sum of its parts. It focuses on the organism in which separate systems and functions are integrated, interdependent, each exerting a profound influence upon all the others. In illness, holism insists that the whole person should be considered rather than the immediate symptoms; it treats the person rather than the disease; it takes into consideration the interplay of physical, emotional, social and environmental aspects of health.

> An holistic approach to health behaviour cautions that it is essential to broaden our perspective on health behaviours beyond those which have become professionally legitimated. The holistic orientation assumes that health is an attribute of individual and group behaviour; its integrity is heightened by its pervasiveness rather than its divisibility.
>
> (Levin *et al.*, 1977)

This wider analysis of health indicates that horizons should extend to areas not usually considered the concern of medicine. Modern illness does not result from decimation by germs, but the ravages of stress and anxiety, contamination by processed foods, and other factors which reduce our resistance to illness. Mitchell (1984) has outlined eight factors she feels are important to health.

1. How much we are exposed to a hazardous environment.
2. How exhausted work inside and outside the home makes us, and how much time and space we have for recuperation.
3. How much money we have.
4. How many worries, and how deep and sustained they are.
5. How hopeful or hopeless we feel.
6. How powerless or powerful we feel.
7. How bored or alienated we feel.
8. How lonely or loved we feel.

When these are examined it is clear that ill health is not just a factor of age. Ageism has transmitted ideas about the inevitability of pain, illness and dependency, and has led to a fear of ageing which in turn has led to neglect, avoidance and the medicalization of the issues. It is essential to develop a non-medical approach to health which involves older people living in a fulfilling retirement, with time for rest and recreation in a clean environment, a reasonable standard of life, freedom from worry, hope for the future, self-confidence and autonomy, and opportunities for friendship, support and intimacy.

If allopathic medicine, with its restricted view of health, has been notably unsuccesful in dealing with the painful and depressing degenerative diseases of old age, there are other directions in which to look. Older people, particularly, can benefit from a holistic approach. Any treatment should begin with the belief that older people are capable of happiness, achievement and health; that each individual is subject to a multitude of different influences; and that it is important to recognize that different personalities, temperaments, emotions and lifestyles all impinge on health. In treating illness, a holistic approach recognizes that the causes of similar illnesses can be quite different, and thus treatment can be based upon an individual diagnosis rather than an universal cure for particular ailments.

Treating the whole person is not a simple task, it being almost impossible for one person to form a complete impression of any other individual, and even more difficult to devise a treatment which corresponds entirely to that individual. The person in the best position to accomplish this is the individual, who needs to be released from the medical constraints which currently prevent this from happening.

5

Escaping the psychology of medical ageism: reasserting personal control

The general conclusion, arising from the survey undertaken in the previous chapter, is that allopathic medicine is important in just one of the factors contributing to ill health, and that even within this, there are questions concerning its efficacy. Yet the importance of the individual within each is self-evident. However, the medicalization of social life has led to a corresponding decrease in personal responsibility. People are told, implicitly, that they can abuse their bodies, and when they break down medicine will be available to pick up the pieces. Abuse your heart, perhaps by bad diet; abuse your lungs, by smoking or breathing polluted air; when they fail, replacements are available. No approach is better suited to encourage individual irresponsibility.

The medical profession has contributed to the undermining of the individual by the 'mystification' of medical care, a process by which specialist knowledge is used to undermine and devalue the general understandings of personal health to which every individual has access. Even natural processes, such as giving birth or dying, have been medicalized. Whenever possible, both are done within the confines of hospital, as if people were no longer capable of undertaking both functions quite adequately with the support of friends. This creates an unnecessary dependence on the holders of medical 'mysteries'. The emergence of medical specialisms, paralleled by the rise of complex drugs and technologies, has created the impression that people are dependent upon those who control them.

Professional mysteries are steadfastly defended. The widespread acceptance of medicine's claim to objective and unchallengeable 'scientific' authority, and to a knowledge which is available only to trained medical professionals, has made people increasingly dependent. The British Medical Association (BMA) does not approve of patients having open access to their medical records, as if health is no longer personal property, and the patient is not to know what is wrong, what is being done, and why. The BMA has also consistently opposed the establishment of an independent complaints system, the suspicion being that its intention is to protect its members from mistakes, misdemeanours, and the problems arising from iatrogenesis.

Yet despite this, there is a steady move back to the 'old' knowledge, some of which almost died through neglect. Alternative medical practice offers less complex, more holistic responses to the maintenance of good health, encouraging self-care, and often self-diagnosis, as the best form of medical treatment. One reason for this has been the poor record of allopathic medicine, particularly in combating non-infectious diseases; but, alongside this, there is a move towards more positive health strategies, which underline the importance of social, economic and political influences on health. This approach actively strives to empower the individual to make genuine, informed decisions about healthy lifestyles (Phillipson and Strang, 1984).

The women's movement has played a central role in this development, struggling against sexist beliefs and practices in medical care that was enabling medicine to assume increasing control over the functioning of the female body, particularly in relation to menstruation, contraception, abortion, pregnancy and childbirth. Attention was focused on the quality of care received by women in a male-dominated medical system, which considered women to be inferior and sickly people, and practised a wide range of physical, psychological and civil abuses upon them. Doyle (1983) outlined two basic medical views of women. First, men were seen as 'normal', and women 'abnormal' in that:

> ... the intellectual, emotional and physical potential of women
> is measured against the male standard and women are found
> to be essentially defective.

Second, the abnormality is seen to arise from the fact that the normal role of women is to reproduce, and that this is the central, determining characteristic of being a woman:

> The capacity to be a mother is no longer seen to make women
> physically ill – just intellectually and emotionally different and
> – by implication – inferior.

The 'well-woman' approach has insisted that women are recognized as normal, healthy individuals. Women have demanded that they have the right to increased knowledge of their anatomy and physiology, and have access to techniques of self-examination. Systematic efforts have been made to demystify medical knowledge, and to bring self-care into primary focus.

Ehrenreich and English (1973) outlined the dual role that medicine played in the life of women. On the one hand, they saw that the medical system, for example, by offering women protection from unwanted pregnancy, was strategic to women's liberation. But they were also clear that medicine was central to the oppression of women. The relations between medicine and old age are similar in that they are capable of both liberating and oppressing. Many analogies exist between the fight that women face to improve the quality and sensitivity of medical services, and the treatment of older people. Whilst medicine has failed to meet women's needs in relation to contraception, abortion, pregnancy and childbirth, older people have been similarly failed in terms of the many wasting, degenerative diseases from which they suffer. Just as menstruation and birth have been seen as an 'illness', and thus legitimate conditions for medical attention, so old age is widely seen as an illness – a terminal one. Whilst women cannot have babies without medical assistance, older people cannot live or, indeed, die without it.

There are more specific analogies. The prescription of tranquillizers has risen alarmingly for both women and older people. Stress and anxiety have become major problems for both groups: for women because they cannot cope with the double burden of work and domestic chores; for older people because of the isolation and boredom of old age. Similarly, the increase of mental illness in women and old people have their origins in social expectations: too much of women, too little of older people. Both groups are controlled by medication, but the underlying basis of their problems remain unresolved. Medicine is a quick and relatively simple solution for doctors, but not for the quality of life of 'patients'.

There is one major difference between the two groups. The women's movement is actively seeking to regain control, and has already achieved significant successes. There is no similar movement for older people, who remain old, ill, and far from in control of their bodies. There is barely the recognition that control is an issue. The medical approach to older people needs to be challenged in line with what is now happening for women.

Reassuming control will involve problematical changes. Resistance to change can arise from three separate quarters. First, there are the ageist assumptions which indicate that change in old age is not possible, or even useful; this is allied to the conservatism of many older people. Then there is the self-interest and convenience of carers. Each needs to be recognized, and the issues tackled.

Human life, regardless of age, is conservative. People will do anything to avoid introducing radical change in their lives. Habits are established whilst young, usually preceding conscious individual thought or action, and so many are culturally transmitted through successive generations. Whilst people do change, and vary their outlook throughout a lifetime, it is often difficult to change habits and ideas which for many years have been considered important.

Ageism suggests that older people become increasingly incapable of change, often based on the premise that if personal decline and death is inevitable, it is pointless to try to prevent it. The element of truth contained in this is extended to explain that older people cannot alter their lifestyle, even if it is damaging their health. The arguments are well known. They have done such things for many years, enjoyed a long life, and are happy living as they do, so why should they change? In any case, does changing the practices of a lifetime have any effect once old age has been reached? The damage to health has surely occurred, so change is pointless, and believing this, older people become resigned to pain, discomfort and illness.

Such attitudes are rooted more in the despair and negativism of ageism than reality. The evidence is that change is never too late, particularly if the objective is not to prevent decline and death, but to prolong a satisfactory quality of life for as long as possible. However, to acquire this requires a positive mental attitude towards life in the later years. If old age becomes miserable it is often the result of life habits which run counter to the maintenance of good health. To accept that older people cannot change is to submit to ageism; it fails to recognize the need for change when change is important to future quality of life. The difficulties of change have to be weighed against the pain, discomfort, incapacity, illness and disease that otherwise accompanies the ageing process.

For the carer, facilitating change also means a considerable commitment which can be avoided by accepting that ageing is a painful experience that has to be endured. It is certainly easier to resort to quick, straightforward allopathic medical intervention as a sufficient response. Dominant attitudes support this view. It is easier to associate a condition with some impersonal cause, perhaps some chance encounter with an itinerant germ, or the ageing process itself. Allopathic medicine sustains this view by providing treatment which imposes no personal cost to favoured lifestyles. The underlying cause of illness is overlooked, colluding with the tendency to rationalize that illness results from misfortune, thus preventing people from taking personal responsibility for their health.

The tendency to rely on experts rather than on ourselves, what we know, and what we feel, is also unhelpful. The prestige of medicine has made many people hesitate to deal with even the mildest health problem. Also, allopathy has made health appear very complicated; and the more complicated the treatment appears, the more impotent the individual feels. Medical terminology, treatment with dangerous toxic drugs, and complex health machinery, have all undermined individual confidence.

Older people have a wide life experience, through which they develop a diversity of needs, strengths and weaknesses; age is just one facet of their complex personalities. Moreover, it is often not a dominant feature in their thinking and behaviour. People of any age can accept change when they recognize the need for it. It is this recognition that creates the dynamic for change, and it involves several prerequisites:

1. Accurate information concerning the nature and cause of illness.
2. Understanding the value and purpose of appropriate lifestyle change.
3. Working through individual feelings about the consequences and difficulties of change.
4. Arriving at new decisions about the way the individual is living.

To enable the development of positive attitudes, change at both an individual and societal level is required. Good health does not just mean freedom from pain or illness, but a positive feeling of vigour and well-being, with continuing social engagement. This is often called a social as opposed to a medical, concept of health. Many older people need convincing about this, and where this is so, counselling is extremely important. Such skills are always useful when working with older people, but never more so when there is a fixed, unchanging, and negative outlook on life (Scrutton, 1989).

The starting point for this new involvement in personal health would be to recognize the natural healing power of the body, and that this is the starting point for bringing back individual control over health.

VIS MEDICATRIX NATURAE: THE HEALING POWER OF NATURE

Animals living in the wild appear to realize that there is nothing complex about health, that it is the outcome of sensible living habits.

On the rare occasions that animals become ill, they seek cover, rest as much as possible, and stop eating. Their objective is simple: to rest until health returns, directing all bodily energies to the task of self-healing. It is this simple recognition that within each organism there is a power which ensures that the heart beats, the blood flows, the lungs breathe, and the brain functions, that humanity seems to have lost. Yet it is these powers that enables us to maintain health, and recover from illness.

Medicalization is central to this loss of knowledge. After illness we often attribute recovery to some form of medication rather than the self-healing powers of the body, which are either taken for granted, or forgotten altogether, but which are capable of dealing satisfactorily with the most serious ailments.

The mechanisms of *vis medicatrix naturae* are so effective that most illness is self-terminating. Cuts and wounds are closed by blood clotting, and healed by passing extra blood to it. Infections are fought by fever, a rise in body temperature which enhances the capacity of the body to defend itself. Our organs and tissues are regularly renewed, our cells cleansed, our blood purified, our digestive system purged. Even when we abuse our bodies, they continue to fight for the renewal of health. The complexity of this operation can be witnessed in something as simple as a minor cut or graze:

> As soon as skin is broken, the body starts . . . forming blood clots to prevent further bleeding, manufacturing fibrin to close the wound. Also, white blood cells, antitoxins and antibiotics are immediately rallied and rushed into concentration at the site of the trauma, where they help to immobilize and destroy the bacteria that have entered the body through the wound, including the dead bacteria. The cells in the area surrounding the wound that have escaped trauma remain undamaged increase their workload by supplying extra oxygen, food and materials for repairing the damaged tissues and building new ones.
>
> (McIntyre, 1987)

The recuperative powers of the body have been described as a homeostatic response, a process that seeks to return the body to its 'normal' state of balance and harmony. Yet it often achieves more than this, leaving the body in a condition better adapted to future challenges. Fractured bones heal making them stronger; scar tissue is better able to resist further damage; recovery from infectious disease gives the body a lasting immunity to reoccurrence. Thus, the self-healing properties of the body enables a permanent adaptation to the challenges of the world.

The best medical care does little more than mobilize these self-healing mechanisms. It has been estimated that about 80% of patients require no treatment at all, and will get better without medical intervention, whilst another 10% of patients require only information and advice (Coleman, 1986a). Our survival depends more upon sophisticated internal biological and psychological mechanisms rather than medical intervention. These enable the organism to adapt to an immense variety of situations that would otherwise threaten our existence. Indeed, our ability to adapt is usually so effective that most challenges to health do not result in illness, and even when they do, our adaptive responses can usually bring about a spontaneous recovery.

Central to the process of providing the body with a natural resistance to disease is the immune system. This system, operated through lymphocytes, part of the lymphatic system which combats invading organisms, neutralizes a wide variety of toxic substances, controls viruses, bacteria, fungi and allergies, and surveys other cells of the body, destroying any which have become malignant or cancerous. The system is delicately tuned and discriminative, being able to discriminate between personal cells, which it accepts, and foreign cells, which it attempts to neutralize or destroy.

Lymph is a colourless fluid, which cleanses body tissue fluid and returns it to the blood. Lymph is absorbed by the tissues through many thread-like capillaries, all eventually connected to a multitude of lymphatic glands, or nodes. These purify the lymph, producing antibodies, antitoxins, and the cells that process the lymph itself. Unlike the blood, lymph has no natural pump, but is kept moving by activity. Sedentary people, especially those who suffer from tension, eating a high-fat, low-fibre diet, are particularly susceptible to blocked lymph nodes. When the lymph stops flowing freely, lymphatic tissues, like the spleen, tonsils and thymus gland, and a multitude of lymph nodes throughout the body, can become inflamed, causing exhaustion or sickness.

The efficiency of the immune system appears to decline with age, making it less able to defend itself. This has led to the hypothesis that the ageing immune system experiences a passive process of wearing out, thereby indicating a close association between the functioning of the immune system, and age-related disease patterns (Adler et al., 1978). With many older people there is certainly a failure to repair cell damage, and an active process of self-destruction as the immune system loses its ability to distinguish between personal and foreign cells, leading to diseases such as cancer and autoimmune diseases, many associated with old age, such as arthritis and pernicious anaemia.

Yet whether this age-related decline in the immune system is caused by ageing itself, or by factors unconnected with age, remains unclear. The immune system is certainly devastated by modern lifestyle, with the number and frequency of autoimmune diseases increasing. Psychoneuroimmunology, a new and controversial area of health research, has made important discoveries which indicate that our state of mind can directly affect the immune system. Its efficiency is reduced by stress, depression, diet, and atmospheric disturbance, at which time its ability to fight illness becomes seriously impaired, quite regardless of age. It is known that there is a two-way pathway between the immune system and the brain, with various hormones acting as messengers. Stress caused by bereavement, and other emotional trauma, has been shown to affect the functioning of the lymphatic system, and the immunity this provides against viruses and the growth of cancer cells. When the immune system under-functions in this way, people are more likely to catch colds, influenza and other infectious diseases (Argyle, 1987).

Thus, factors which commonly impinge upon the lives of older people can play an important role in the effectiveness of the immune system, as much as ageing itself. Body chemicals that influence emotions and the ability to feel pain interact directly with the immune system. The link between immunity, ageing and health seems to be interwoven in a complex pattern, the one relating to, and being affected by, the others.

The therapeutic success of many 'non-medical' healers, such as faith healing, Zen, yoga and others, should be re-evaluated in the light of the body's self-healing capacity, and their validity reassessed according to their ability to enhance the natural recuperative powers of the body rather than their scientific credibility.

Similarly, the action of allopathic medicine needs to be questioned, for the effect of surgery and toxic drugs can actually inhibit the process of self-healing. Allopathy, by definition, introduces into the body substances which provoke a conflicting, or opposite condition. This can lead to the body becoming lazy, relying upon drugs rather than natural internal mechanisms to achieve the task. One example is the treatment of constipation by laxatives, known to reduce the body's own natural propensity to empty the bowel when taken over long periods. Steroidal drug treatment of arthritis and asthma is another, these reproducing the action of naturally occurring corticosteroids. Whilst their powerful impact can suppress uncomfortable symptoms quickly, they can also reduce the natural production of steroids so that the body eventually becomes unable to respond in the normal way. The drug designed to make the body better can, in this way, increase its vulnerability to disease.

There are theories of medicine which present an alternative view of illness, and its treatment. Most are based on the premise that natural processes within the body will maintain health. Naturopathy represents the purist expression of this holistic view, stating that whilst the healing process can be aided, it must never be thwarted, checked or suppressed. It believes that no one who is healthy inside can become a victim of bacterial or viral infection, that disease emanates from within the body, the predisposing factor being lowered vitality within a body clogged with waste materials and impurities.

Treatment for fever illustrates the differences between the two approaches. Naturopaths interpret fever as a response to acute disease, an example of a natural healing response, with microorganisms acting as beneficial agents. The purpose of the fever is to rid the body of the toxins and impurities arising from unhealthy living habits. When these superficial manifestations of disease are suppressed by medical drugs, naturopaths believe that whilst the patient appears to get well, it is at the cost of more serious and lasting chronic disease appearing in later years.

Allopathic medicine treats the symptoms of illness. The 'germ' theory of disease typifies this approach. Germs are seen as 'the enemy', their activity during illness an indication that they are the causal factor. When Pasteur elaborated his celebrated theory of disease it was welcomed as the final proof of this approach, from which solutions to all disease would eventually be forthcoming. Yet even Pasteur began to understand the true relationship of germs to disease late in his career, when he stated that, 'The germ is nothing, the soil is everything, by which he meant that germs thrive only in a suitable environment (Trattler, 1985).

Naturopaths believe that the error of allopathic medicine has been to assume that as germs are present and active when disease is present, they are the cause of disease. Their interpretation of the function of germs is quite different, seeing them as part of the natural forces enlisted by the body to fight the illness. The body is always full of germs. Naturopaths believe that they are discovered alongside disease because these are bodily mechanisms used to break down and eliminate accumulated toxic matter. Germs are present in disease not as the cause, but as the body's agent seeking to eliminate the real cause of disease, toxicity.

Certainly, not everyone exposed to germs becomes ill. The most striking demonstration of this was given by Dr Pettenkofer in the nineteenth century who, before a class of students, swallowed sufficient cholera germs to kill a regiment of soldiers. He believed that within a healthy body, natural immunity would prevent harmful bacteria from gaining a foothold.

> Germs are of no account in cholera. The important thing is the disposition of the individual.
>
> (Benjamin, 1961)

Natural healing insists that germs should not be destroyed, as this only suppresses disease until it returns later in more chronic forms. Drugs complicate illness by interfering with the natural chemistry of the body, suppressing rather than curing disease, pushing it deeper into the body. Thus, whilst drugs can appear to improve health in the short term, they can ultimately lead to more serious, chronic disease.

This is because drug treatment is believed to interfere with natural body chemistry, undermining the function of the body's natural immunity, and eventually increasing susceptibility to illness and disease. If naturopathy is correct, the impact of drug treatment is to suppress disease only for it to re-emerge later in life. The experience of many older people supports this view. Sickness, such as colds and influenza, apparently cured or ameliorated by medical drugs, reappear after a few months, often in a stronger, more virulent form, perhaps as bronchitis or pneumonia. Even antibiotics are now recognized as a two-edged sword. They do deal with infections; but they also weaken the ability of the immune defence system dealing with further encounters, and they also kill off helpful bacteria in the body. Naturopathic medicine suggests that the suppression of acute illness results in delayed iatrogenic effects, taking the form of gout, arthritis, arteriosclerosis, cancer, and other chronic conditions which would not have developed if earlier illness had been allowed to run its natural course, or were avoided by a healthier lifestyle.

In contrast, recovery from illness using alternative forms of treatment is usually slower, but once recovered the individual actually feels stronger. There are two reasons for this. By bolstering the general health and efficiency of weak organs or systems, alternative medicine increases resistance to further illness, and prevents the development of chronic disease. Perhaps more important is the general advice about lifestyle and other factors that usually accompanies treatment. These may have initially caused the illness, and if they remain unmodified, can lead to its reoccurrence.

Which interpretation, allopathic or naturopathic, is correct is clearly a crucial question. Certainly, the two explanations are so diametrically

73

opposed that the recent trend of describing 'alternative' therapies as 'complementary' is difficult to accept. It is hardly 'complementary' if allopathy seeks to kill germs, whereas naturopathy, and many other holistic medical systems, seeks to support and assist them.

Most older people have learnt for decades that illness is caused by pathogens. If this is incorrect, it might explain why comprehensive schemes of allopathic medicine have led to more, rather than less, illness, and why chronic disease is increasing rapidly. The idea that health and illness is closely connected to the way life is experienced and lived, and that there are alternative explanations and treatments for illness, will be a revelation for many people.

Yet this realization can be more beneficial than this, helping eventually to develop the belief that it is possible, even for older people, to rely upon self-help in the maintenance of health. Certainly, it is not appropriate to rely entirely on the immune system for health, particularly as we grow older, for it is clear that many factors in modern life undermine and thwart our capacity to stay well. We all have to be able to help ourselves, to actively participate in decisions which relate to the maintenance of health.

SELF-HELP

It is possible to be ageing and healthy and, perhaps more important, to be in control. Self-help is vital. There is no more depressing condition than for older people to feel that they are not in control of their lives. Dependence, with its association with depression, and the effect this has on health, represents an unhappy circularity too often associated with old age.

Self-help requires individuals to know more about their health, and the reasons for it, than dominant medical opinion allows. Like animals, we have health instincts which can help overcome the effects of illness, and recognize some direct relationships between certain practices and the alleviation of symptoms. The individual can determine how best to maintain health; we experience our condition, and feel the symptoms directly. Doctors can only question and observe; the most useful basis of medical diagnosis is dependent upon information given by the individual. Nor is diagnosis always straightforward, for some conditions such as pain, depression and, perhaps old age itself, do not submit to physical tests which can confirm or deny their existence.

Yet self-help is limited by two important factors. The first concerns our knowledge of illness and what is available to put it right, compounded by our lack of self-confidence in the validity of personal insights. The second concerns the impact of illness itself, which thwarts the ability to function properly, impairing the judgement of the most resilient individuals, undermining confidence about what is happening, and what should be done. These uncertainties drive people to the doctor in search of expert diagnosis and cure. We feel ill, we want the doctor to remove our worst fears, and make us better. This situation places both parties under pressure: patients want reassurance and doctors are expected to find instant solutions. Neither expectation is particularly realistic or helpful.

This pattern is particularly important for older people, given the general fears about dependency and long-term illness. All sick people tend to be less assertive, more compliant, more willing to delegate responsibility for their health. Moreover, they abrogate responsibility in proportion to the degree of pain, or the closeness of death. Many people, either through fear or lack of knowledge, become debilitated by health problems: even mild conditions can appear to signify a serious health problem.

Allopathic medicine does not ignore the benefits of self-help, but its commitment is usually limited to basic advice about personal lifestyle factors. Self-care is a broader concept in which individual responsibility includes sharing with the doctor the process of diagnosis, and the choice and application of treatment. Four aspects of self-care have been identified by Levin *et al.*, (1977): health maintenance, disease prevention, self-diagnosis and self-treatment. This involves decision-making, self-observation, symptom perception and labelling, judgement of severity, and choice and assessment of treatment options, as well as making health professionals accountable to patients.

Older people, and their carers, should seek to develop a partnership with doctors, rather than the more usual master/servant relationship – one which recognizes both the limitations and strengths of medical intervention. Yet assuming control over personal health means doing more than democratizing health-care relationships. It requires the dissemination of knowledge about the nature of health and illness, empowering individuals to ask questions, and make decisions on the basis of that knowledge. Medical resistance to this is considerable. Patients often leave surgeries with unasked, or unanswered, questions, not only because the doctor's time is limited, but because there is general disapproval based on a feeling that it is inappropriate for untrained people to question medical professionals.

The almost exclusive concept of professional health intervention has . . . . . deflected interest in lay interventions by encouraging the view that such practices are dangerous, scientifically unsubstantiated, and associated with superstitious and parochial mentalities. In effect, this view holds that self-care in health is a folk practice, culture-bound and 'indigenous', riddled with absurd and ineffectual remedies, rampantly empirical, contributing on occasion to unnecessary delays in seeking professional care and often implicated in the failure of laypersons to follow prescribed medical regimens. Self-care, so viewed, is considered a vestigial or at best a residual health function in the wake of the growth of 'modern medicine' and is to be avoided and deplored.

(Levin *et al.*, 1977)

This reluctance is based on social and economic factors which underlay the status of the medical profession, which treats illness within the profitable health-care industry by selling complex drugs, sophisticated screening programmes, and other high-technology products. This technology is difficult to share, and there is usually little interest in doing so. Medicine too often involves complicated treatment which frequently obscures the simpler answers which lay within personal reach.

What most of us know about health is that which the medical profession is prepared to tell us. What is known arises either from our experience of medical practice, or what we are told of its achievements. We learn that illness is caused by germs, that treatment involves identifying the disease, understanding its pathology, and attacking the cause. Yet it is important for older people to be freed from a medical ideology which intimates that to be old is to be sick, and that to be sick is to be dependent upon medical professionals. This becomes possible only through the development of increased knowledge and understanding of the issues involved.

With the aid of a concerted educational programme, there is an increasing conviction that most diseases can be prevented without medical assistance. Self-care can be important in preventing, treating, and stabilizing the most prevalent and debilitating illnesses. Contrary to public perception, the causes of many modern illnesses, such as arthritis, most cancers, heart attacks and strokes, are known, and health maintenance is relatively straightforward, attainable without the use of drugs or, indeed, any form of medical intervention.

The objective of self-help is to increase the coping ability of the individual both in terms of knowledge and confidence. Sick people often wish to do something constructive to prevent or cope with illness, and this positive approach can be medically helpful. Even when self-care is inappropriate, or when an individual wishes to be passive, evidence indicates that better communication and mutual understanding between physician and patient facilitates patient recovery (Levin *et al.*, 1977). Everything that follows is an exploration of the ways in which the individual can act in relation to their own health.

THE PSYCHOLOGY OF ILLNESS

Optimistic, happy people are known to become ill less often, and less seriously, than those who are regularly unhappy, anxious and pessimistic. The benefit of positive expectations in old age can be seen in studies outlining the importance of psychosomatic illness, the placebo effect, the power of suggestion, and faith healing, all examples of the power of the mind over physical illness.

The impact of emotions, such as tension, fear, anxiety, sadness and depression, is often to debilitate the body. Migraine, ulcers, digestive problems, even chronic backache, cancer and heart disease are now thought to be related to our emotional lives. Conversely, smiling, laughter, happiness and optimism promote relaxation, and reduce the likelihood of contracting stress-related illness.

Yet the potential health benefits of positive mental attitudes have to be contrasted with the negative, ageist perceptions that depresses so many older people. Old age is not generally considered a time of happiness or optimism, but one dominated by negative feelings, attitudes and emotions. The association between ageing, depression and illness is probably closer than realized; ageist expectations can probably result in the very illnesses that older people fear.

Depression is too often the companion of old age, and can prove to be as debilitating as any disease. It increases the speed of the ageing process, and makes the prospect of old age less acceptable than it might otherwise be. Depression is a significant disease, with multiple causes rooted in the social experience of the individual. Its symptoms are sadness, tearfulness, sleep disturbance, loss of appetite, neglect of appearance, fearfulness, anxiety, indecision, mood changes, tiredness and weakness, poor concentration, loss of memory, and loss of libido and sociability.

Nor is depression just a mental state. Illness and pain can result from emotional states. Selye (1956) first demonstrated how exhaustion can be caused by frustration or suppressed rage, detailing the negative effects these emotions have on body chemistry. More recent evidence has confirmed that the mind plays a decisive role in illness, and that a peaceful mind leads to a healthier body. Considerable physical and mental illness can result from chronic unhappiness, anxiety, pessimism, tension and conflict.

Depression is related to the common social experience of ageing. Retirement, and the loss of social relationships and status can lead to lowered self-esteem and decreased interest in life, important contributors to depression, and thus illness. The loss of close friends and relatives, either through divorce and bereavement, is known to increase the ri⁻¹ of illness. People can die of a broken heart, as so often demonstrated by the frequency with which one life-long partner dies shortly after the other, even when the individual is apparently healthy.

Older people need to learn to cope with their fears about illness. Hypochondriasis, an excessive preoccupation with health, is more common in later life. The tension produced by fear can restrict the flow of blood, hormones and nutrients to the body, which can itself generate illness. Health is best served not by increased anxiety, but by the optimism arising from the maintenance of satisfactory social and emotional lifestyle. Purpose, and the will to live, are important considerations for older people. Hopefulness and optimism can help to maintain purposiveness and immunity.

There is evidence that a positive attitude helps to produce a healthier body. A study of health statistics undertaken by one of the largest health insurers in the United States of America indicated that people who practise some form of meditation seek less health care, and become ill less than half as often as other people. There is also evidence suggesting that positive thinking produces good health. Happiness and contentment make a significant difference to health, with happier people having greater immunity from illness (Gidley and Shears, 1988; Argyle 1987; Cousins, 1979). It is also possible for older people to react positively to stress-related illness. It has been indicated in psychosomatics that their emotions can alter their endocrine balance, impair their blood supply and blood-pressure, impede their digestion, change their body temperature, and produce a sustained state of emotional stress causing physiological changes that lead to disease (Cheraskin *et al.*, 1974).

Likewise, biofeedback, the technique of learning the voluntary control of internal states, has been shown to enable the regulation of body temperature, heartbeat, brain-wave rate, and even mood and emotion. This ability is available to everyone, and developing the ability offers some potentially powerful applications for self-healing. Headaches and migraine are probably related to high levels of tension, and to restricted flow of blood to the brain, so biofeedback can be particularly important in this respect with such ailments (Carlson, 1975).

Although the problem of scientific proof is considerable, such a connection between the mind and health should not be surprising with so many connections between the conscious and unconscious processes of the brain, and every organ in the body.

There is also evidence that smiling and laughter are not just social gestures, but have an effect on the maintenance of health. The benefits of smiling and laughter were first outlined by the French psychologist, Israel Waynbaum, who became convinced that by using the facial muscles, hormonal mechanisms in the brain were activated which sent chemical messages throughout the body (Hodgkinson, 1987). The zygomatic, or 'smile' muscle increases blood supply to the brain, affecting the production of certain hormones, and directly influencing the rate the heart beats and blood-pressure. Laughter helps to increase oxygen flow to the lungs, deepens breathing, and aids circulation. Smiling and laughter also relaxes us, lightens our overall mood, and makes us feel happy.

Moreover, it is the physical process of smiling and laughter that is beneficial, not the actual feelings. Smile therapy operates on the principle of 'first expression, then the emotion'. The physical action of smiling can help depressed and unhappy people feel better, thereby breaking the vicious circle of unhappiness, illness, misery and further illness.

The most notable exponent of this therapy is Norman Cousins (Cousins, 1979), who confounded his doctors by recovering from ankylosing spondylitis, an 'incurable' illness in which the spine becomes increasingly immobile, crippling the patient progressively with pain. He did so by hiring films that made him laugh.

Laughing affects every organ in the body, and the bigger the belly laugh, the better it is for us. When we laugh we secrete hormones that stimulate the heart and act as natural painkillers. Stress is reduced. Calories are burned off and digestion is improved.

(Hodgkinson, 1987)

It was calculated that when Cousins laughed for 10 minutes, it gave him an anaesthetic effect which lasted two hours. Emotions are known to affect the secretion of hormones, especially from the thyroid and adrenal glands. The brain and pituitary gland contain a group of hormones callecd endorphins, antidepressant chemicals created naturally within the body, which react physiologically like morphine, heroin, and other opiate substances, and which relieve pain by acting on the source of pain itself, but also by inhibiting the emotional response (suffering) usually associated with pain. In this way, mental attitudes can affect the secretion of endorphin, and thereby the perception of pain and disease. Despite Cousins' recovery, and the supporting evidence surrounding the general theory, the medical reaction was predictably dismissive, although the idea is gradually finding interest and recognition.

The placebo effect indicates that whilst drugs are not always necessary for recovery, belief in recovery is. It is now widely accepted that interest in life, and the will to live, combats disease. Cancer patients who resist the disease are known to increase their chances of survival over those who passively accept it, or who succumb to fear. Many illnesses, including cancer, frequently strike after a major bereavement or loss, when our emotions have the greatest impact on our immune resistance to disease.

Experiments in hypnosis and meditation indicate that individuals are capable of influencing their immunity to illness through controlling the immunological cells contained within the blood supply. The argument is that if the psyche can damage the immune system, it can also be used positively to support it. The idea of visualization, using mental imagery to boost the immune system, can encourage patients to imagine their immune systems playing an active, aggressive role in attacking foreign cells in their bodies, and this has been found helpful in reinforcing recovery from certain illnesses.

Such evidence supports the idea that individuals can use their mental power to influence recovery. The implication is that older people should make themselves happy by smiling, or finding ways of encouraging laughter. Certainly, smiling and laughter have no side-effects; happiness is an entirely safe tranquillizer, with the additional benefit of assisting companionship and social life.

If older people could lead, and be helped to lead, more contented lives, they would increase their chances of maintaining health. There are many other antidotes to depression: the simply enjoyment arising from buying new clothes, changing hairstyle, a good holiday, relaxing and forgetting about urgent matters, can all be helpful.

Yet, perhaps the most natural cure for depression is exercise, the chemical benefits of which is to stimulate the production of endorphins. The elation reported by many athletes following exercise is believed to be the result of this. The benefits of exercise are readily available to older people, although the opportunities for exercise, and the recognition of the need for exercise in old age, is perhaps less well developed. The benefits of exercise are considered more fully in Chapter 8.

6

Maintaining social engagement: combating loneliness and loss

Human beings are gregarious animals, with most aspects of our lives spent in close, often intimate interdependence with other people. The family, the maintenance of friends and daily companionship, are the basis for an active, stimulating involvement in life. This dynamic interaction with other people is very important; it is perhaps not an exaggeration to say that our very existence depends on having other people to love and care for, and to be loved and cared for in return.

Throughout life the number of friends we lose, either through social mobility, accident or death, gradually increases, making older people particularly prone to loneliness and loss. Ageing people find that they have a reducing circle of friends, so those remaining are of longer-standing, and increasing significance. Each loss becomes more difficult to overcome. A state of deep emotional deprivation can be the result of a serious loss of strong emotional attachments. Avoiding isolation, and replacing lost friends and partners is always possible, but with ageing it requires increasing effort and determination.

Friendship is important at all stages of life. Younger people, when faced with sensory deprivation arising from a lack of social and emotional stimulation, begin to show signs of apathy, memory loss, mental confusion, and even mental illness. Many older people live in circumstances close to solitary confinement, their days filled with monotonous and meaningless routine, interminable evenings, and lonely nights. It is not surprising that similar personality breakdown and mental deterioration can result.

Ensuring that life is full, active and stimulating is not straight-forward. Many factors other than ageing reduce the social oppor-tunities of older people, resulting in loneliness and isolation. These range from retirement, reduced income, bereavement, reduced mobility, disengagement, cultural change or social mobility. Hearing difficulty which affects many older people, is another isolating condition. The implication is that decline in old age results not from lack of potential, but takes place when abilities are not sufficiently utilized.

Yet even if loss in old age is unavoidable, it is not loss itself but the way older people face up to loss that is important. The most effective way of preventing social and mental deterioration through loneliness is for the individual to face up to it, accept that it is their responsibility, to make new friends, and to adopt new hobbies and interests. The worst response is to become depressed. Self-pity rather than positive action can arise from isolation, leading to ideas of being left alone, neglected or forsaken. Life is not fair; life is not forever; it has to be lived, regardless of the circumstances. The most debilitating result of loss is the feeling that there is no future opportunity or hope, no chance of satisfactorily replacing loss.

Socially inactive and isolated older people are likely to be increasingly unhappy, bored and unfulfilled. Lack of social stimulation can cause mental and physical skills to decline rapidly, leading to passivity, apathy and lethargy. A vicious circularity follows when a decline in alertness, and reduced interest in life, leads to further loss of interest in regaining entry into social life. The chronic cycle of low activity, increased stress, social withdrawal and mental depression is common to many older people.

Illness can result from the unhappiness that accompanies declining physical, mental and social involvement. Older people need to continue using their minds and bodies in order to retain their agility and health. Gore (1973) calls for an expansionist rather than a reductionist attitude towards life, an approach which allows older people to exercise and retain their potential vitality. She stresses that to remain active and independent involves considerable effort, requiring regular questioning and adapting of attitudes, habits and activities.

Many carers do not try to break this cycle. They feel that they might invade the right of older people to privacy and self-determination. Some suggest that older people have a right to 'disengage'. Whilst this is so, it is a view which is also an easier option than actively encouraging social reintegration.

These negative views are supported by ageist assumptions that relates social apathy with the process of ageing. Disengagement theory is the most well-known exposition of this. The theory, first postulated by Cummings and Henry (1961) has served to justify the experience of isolation and loneliness in old age. Its key argument is that ageing people deliberately choose to withdraw from social involvement. It presents old age as a separate, distinct stage of life, interpreting behaviour to suggest that older people no longer find social involvement satisfying. In doing so, they established older people as a homogeneous group which was unwilling to participate in mainstream social functions.

> Ageing is an inevitable mutual withdrawal or disengagement resulting in decreased interaction between the ageing person and others in the social system he belongs to. The process may be initiated by the individual or by others in the situation. The aged person may withdraw more markedly from some classes of people while remaining relatively close to others. His withdrawal may be accompanied from the outset by an increased preoccupation with himself; certain institutions in society may make the withdrawal easy for him. When the aging process is complete the equilibrium which existed in middle life between the individual and his society has given way to a new equilibrium characterized by a greater distance and an altered type of relationship.
>
> (Cummings and Henry, 1961)

The theory has legitimized the exclusion of older people from the social and economic world, and whilst it may now be discredited in academic quarters, its widespread social influence remains. Old age is commonly seen by many people, young and old, as a time of withdrawal from all forms of social involvement. Its influence is still evident in many popular books on old age; Stoppard (1983) appears to accept the phenomenon when she states that 'most of us begin to withdraw from the social whirl through choice', and goes on to discuss this as if it was a normal rather than a structural reaction to growing old.

Indeed, withdrawal for many older people can seem to offer a means of liberation from the stresses and tensions of social life. For those engaged in the toil of daily living, retirement and withdrawal can appear to be attractive propositions. The family has been raised, a pension is available, and the main duties of life are complete. The future offers the prospect of quiet contemplation, the pursuit of hobbies in peace and tranquillity, the ability to travel, to fulfil old dreams, or just to enjoy spending time relaxing with friends.

There are two main problems with this view of peaceful, disengaged old age. For most older people, the reality is quite different. Social alienation brings with it a multitude of emotional, social and economic problems, placing older people in an aimless world on the fringes of mainstream society, with loneliness, isolation and depression a central feature of life.

However, the main failure of disengagement theory is its inability to distinguish between human activity that is freely chosen and actively desired by the individual, and action that is socially constructed and structurally enforced. The theory links human behaviour entirely with personal volition, discounting the constraints of dominant social attitudes and values, which structure the lives and expectations of older people. Such theories:

> ... simply provide a convenient rationalization for unequal power relationships, presenting as 'natural and inevitable' something which is merely expedient. From its inception, disengagement theory attracted a highly critical response. The concept itself was seen as legitimating a form of social redundancy among the old, a product of structural changes in the economy and the labour market.
>
> (Fennel *et al.*, 1988)

Disengagement theory ignores the existence of structural pressures which produce conformity to the elderly stereotype. Retirement is the clearest example of socially constructed disengagement. Retirement is often presented as a feature of modern philanthropy, a recognition that the individual has contributed sufficiently to economic life, with retirement the reward for past services. Yet whilst not denying that many people find retirement a positive and welcome experience, altering their focus from work to the family and outside interests, for most older people, especially those who found work fulfilling, or whose retirement was accompanied by a significant loss of income and status, retirement is a negative experience. Most retirees will identify with Shakespeare's King Lear, who gave up his lands and power to his daughters, trusting that thereafter they would care for him. Yet, once divested of his social status and role, Lear was treated with disdain, no longer able to command the respect due to his former status.

Employment provides a number of hidden benefits, often unnoticed until given up. Work structures the use of time, provides shared experiences and social contacts outside the family, links the individual to broader goals and purposes, gives status and a sense of identity, and provides a raised level of activity (Argyle, 1987). Employment also confirms personal competence and worth, both to ourselves and others. Living on social welfare, or even on savings or occupational pensions, seems to many to be an impersonal, humiliating experience, accentuating growing uselessness and dependence. These feelings are often reinforced by demographic arguments, which indicate an increasing proportion of 'unproductive' retired people are a burden requiring support from a reducing working population.

These ageist perceptions do little to confirm social philanthropy. Philanthropy becomes a stick with which to beat older people; they are obliged not to work, and are then castigated for being a burden. Social respect continues to depend largely on current social role and achievement. Past accomplishment, as Lear found, is quickly discounted. Retired people are attributed status according to social attitudes dominated by the 'production-oriented' values of capitalism. Retired people do not produce wealth, so they lose respect in a world which appraises personal value in terms of productivity. Retirement in this sense is not a privilege; it becomes demoralizing, stripping the individual of his or her social role, status and self-esteem.

The sole justification for retirement is chronological age, not ability to work. The skills and knowledge of older people, developed over a lifetime, are rejected. The pressures, tensions, and rate of change of modern social life are used to discount the social and economic contribution that older people can make. Retirement contributes to feelings of personal diminution. Many older people feel marginalized, stigmatized, isolated, unloved, ignored and personally devalued. Former social channels are removed when there is no workplace to attend, and no circle of colleagues with whom to socialize. Enforced retirement not only restricts social contact, but often results in some withdrawal from friendships with employed people, often because they cannot afford the costs of socialization.

Enforced retirement ensures that those wishing to continue their working life are thrust into what can become a depressing idleness. Unemployment can lead to apathy and boredom if people find that they cannot organize their time. Social life can become unattractive if many former pastimes and opportunities are barred through loss of income, loss of physical or mental health or, indeed, through social discouragement. Endless leisure becomes demoralizing if there is nothing to offer stimulation. Long periods of idleness leads to many unsatisfactory adjustments, such as killing time by staying in bed late, or watching television, smoking or drinking.

There is no evidence to support the ageist assumption that older people cannot continue to be socially and physically active. It is often the assumption itself that becomes self-fulfilling. If older people demand less of themselves, and fail to maintain interests and skills, or if they become content with lower expectations, decreasing social involvement and achievement can result.

The process can jeopardize health and vitality, reducing the chances of a rewarding, independent and longer life. Research indicates that a high degree of activity, in a specific social role, is positively related to happiness and healthy social adjustments (Fennel *et al.*, 1988). Conversely, increasing loneliness, boredom and dissatisfaction ultimately leads to unhappiness, despair and illness. Many older people respond to low social expectations by losing confidence, self-esteem and, ultimately, their health. Death through illness and suicide is all too common in the period immediately following retirement, often arising from a lack of interest in life itself.

The link between happiness and health is particularly strong for older people. The greatest happiness arises from marriage, and other close, confiding and supportive relationships. The quality of the relationship, measured by the amount of mutual affection and intimacy, is the main source of satisfaction, increasing self-esteem, suppressing negative emotions, and providing support and shared social activities. Many studies have shown that these factors can act as a buffer against physical illness (Argyle, 1987).

Withdrawal from social activity disengages both the body and mind. The problem of social disengagement is not the lack of opportunity for meeting new people, but can arise when older people begin to neglect their personal needs and appearance. If older people no longer see themselves as useful, valuable, contributing members of society, disengagement becomes easier. Older people then adopt unhealthy life habits: overeating and becoming obese; and loneliness leading to drinking and smoking; all of which arise from social isolation.

An agile mind benefits from active participation in social life, just as an agile body needs the regular stimulation of physical exercise. Social involvement exercises the mind, encourages physical activity, and helps to prevent mental decline and depression. The maintenance of health through happiness in old age is enhanced by preserving the harmony shared with family, friends, links with community life, maintaining personal identity, and many other social outlets important to the individual. People who live alone tend to age faster than those who live with other people. Lonelieness is a progressive condition; isolated people have less opportunity to communicate, and eventually they tend to stop reading, thinking, or attempting to socialize. Their increasing introversion can lead to their minds deteriorating through disuse.

For a healthy view of ageing it is fundamental to appreciate that physiological potential exists throughout life. Our potential enables us to respond to physiological challenges, to repair injuries and damage, to improve our performance and to increase our vigour through training, by calling our innate resources into play.

(Gore, 1973)

By remaining socially active older people can help to preserve their mental vitality. Contrary to popular ageist perceptions, the brain does not deteriorate significantly with ageing, but it is important to understand that intellectual performance is maintained by regular 'social' exercise. How this is done is immaterial. Individuals can keep in touch with contemporary social life by joining clubs or groups, involving themselves in creative hobbies, such as gardening or handicrafts, study courses, supporting local sports teams, inviting friends and acquaintances to their home, or by taking holidays. It is possible for everyone to find something that will result in rewarding social involvement.

Increasing numbers of older people are now forming groups to fight their own, age-related issues. Although membership remains small, the trend is important. Too many older people passively accept ageist social roles. Britain is now following the lead of the 'Grey' movement in the USA, with such groups as the Pensioners' Protection Party, the Association of Retired Persons, the British Pensioner and Trades Union Action Association, the Pensioners' Rights Campaign, and Pensioners' Voice (some working under the umbrella organization, the Pensioners' Liaison Forum), all doing valuable work in campaigning for the rights of older people, whilst at the same time keeping themselves active, engaged and healthy.

PERSONALITY FACTORS AND HEALTH

Individual responses to the problems and stresses of life are a reflection of personality. There are people who tend to be consistently happy and optimistic, regardless of difficult events and situations, just as others remain pessimistic and depressed. Although difficult to prove, there are strong links between health and personality, particularly the ageing personality.

There are popular assumptions suggesting that personality is a fixed and unchanging entity. For older people, this is reinforced by ageist presumptions that the ageing personality is particularly inflexible. There is truth in this suggestion; the older personality can become increasingly more of what they have been. Underlying personality tends to remain constant throughout life, and the way people age, whether with self-pity or with tenacity, confirms that people remain what they have always been, often more emphatically so.

Yet both ideas need to be challenged. Personal responses to situations and events are more under individual control than generally recognized. Anxious people can relax; withdrawn people can socialize; unhappy people can be pro-active in creating happiness for themselves.

Individuals tend consistently to choose certain moods because they interpret or cope with situations in characteristic or habitual ways, or because they choose to avoid certain kinds of situation. Extroverts will spend more time in social situations than introverts, and will be less likely to disengage in old age. People pursue situations that tend to confirm their personality traits and motivations, but it remains possible for the individual to choose rewarding rather than unrewarding situations, to decide to be optimistic instead of pessimistic, and to remain involved in situations which maintain social involvement and self-esteem.

> The ageing person continues to exercise choice and to select from the environment in accordance with his own long-established needs. He ages according to a pattern that has a long history and that maintains itself, with adaptation, to the end of life ... There is considerable evidence that in normal men and women, there is no sharp discontinuity of personality with age, but instead an increasing consistency. Those characteristics that have been central to the personality seem to become even more clearly delineated ...
>
> (Neugarten, 1969)

Certain personality types have been associated with diseases, especially those related to stress, such as migraine, asthma, arthritis, heart disease and cancer. The link between personality and disease was first suggested in relation to coronary heart disease in the 1930s. 'Type A' personalities are driven by intense ambition, competitive drive, and a constant preoccupation with deadlines, and are impatient with delays, time-conscious, irritable and aggressive. 'Type B' personalities have a low sense of urgency, and a more phlegmatic attitude towards life. Of the two, 'Type A' personalities were found to be more likely to contract heart disease (Ashton and Davies, 1986).

Cancer victims are frequently described as exceptionally fine, thoughtful, gentle, uncomplaining people; whilst underneath harbouring feelings of unworthiness and self-dislike, and feelings of hostility are bottled up and repressed. This has led to proposals for a 'Type C', or 'cancer', personality. The common features are a tendency to be resentful and unforgiving, an inability to express anger, compliance, conformity, lack of assertiveness, and patience. They tend to become highly aroused by stress, and are less able to release tensions. They have a tendency towards hopelessness, self-pity, depression, a marked inability to form and maintain meaningful relationships, and low self-image (Carlson, 1975; Argyle, 1987).

Personality does not, however, need to be a fixed entity, particularly if it is contributing to chronic illness. If an individual with 'Type A' personality wishes to change in order to overcome heart disease, Friedman and Ulmer (1985) discuss ways in which this can be achieved, based upon personal self-appraisal, and developing a new set of personal 'freedoms'. These include the freedom to overcome insecurity and regain self-esteem; to give and receive love; to take pleasure in friends and family; to recall past life with satisfaction; to listen, play and enjoy tranquillity.

If personality determines the type of illness people are likely to suffer, it is life-style that decides the level of risk, and stress levels that precipitate the outcome (Hope, 1989). The main link between personality and health is through health-related behaviours, which are the coping behaviours by which people react to anxiety and stress. Smoking causes lung cancer, drinking causes alcoholism, over-eating leads to obesity and increases the likelihood of heart disease. Heavy smoking and the consumption of large amounts of animal fats increase our risks of falling victim to illness, with some personality types being more susceptible than others. People have been found to be most at risk when subject to certain kinds of stress, retirement, redundancy, bereavement and similar traumas (Hope, 1989).

Ultimately, the art of reaching a healthy old age is a personalized path towards self-awareness. Old age remains a personal responsibility. There is a tendency to feel that older people should be excused personal faults. If they are aggressive, obsessive, boring, self-centred or hypochondriac, it is excused by their age. They cannot help it. The message should be that they can, and should, be told that they can still do harm, can still change, and make amends. There are many paths to a fulfilling old age. People age differently, and respond to situations differently. Life satisfaction can be gained in many ways. Some will resist ageing, fight every symptom of illness, maintain a high level of social activity, replace lost relationships, and introduce new goals to their lives. Others will succumb to social pressure, living quietly, and disengaging from all but an active involvement in family life, or developing special interests. Even those who 'disengage' completely can accept and adapt to their shrinking world by finding satisfaction in contemplative, or low-activity lives.

GENDER DIFFERENCES

There are also gender-based assumptions concerning the needs of men and women, many related to health which were largely ignored until the work of Finch and Groves (1982), Walker (1983), and Evers (1985), which merit some separate consideration, particularly in relation to older women.

Women generally feel that to admit to ill-health is stigmatizing. Evers (1985) found that women living alone tended to claim that their health was good, despite having many specific health problems. The reason is probably that whilst both sexes subscribe to the view that old age is a time of illness, women's sex-role stereotyping often leads to feelings of guilt or shame at not being able to continue functioning normally. There are two main reasons.

First, women's background in managing the home sanctions greater expectations that they will continue to manage for longer, and under more adverse circumstances than men. There would appear to be no retirement age from household management, with many women being reluctant to relinquish their household and family care tasks.

Second, surveys indicate that the nature of illness suffered by men and women are different. Women endure more painful and disabling conditions, such as arthritis, which develop slowly over longer periods. These become accepted as a 'normal' part of life, and so become regarded less seriously, and with lower priority. Men tend to suffer from life-threatening diseases, such as heart and chest diseases, which arise quickly, are given more priority, and receive greater attention.

It has been found that professional staff often impose these perceptions on their clients, resulting in care strategies which differ fundamentally between men and women. The worst offenders in this respect are often female carers, who expect older women to continue functioning within the home much longer, and under greater pressure than men.

Women use medical services more than men. They visit doctors more often, take more medication, are admitted to hospital more often, and are more frequently diagnosed as having psychiatric problems. The reason is perhaps that the sick role can liberate, providing women with a welcome chance to withdraw from everyday pressures. After a lifetime of caring for others, illness presents an opportunity for women to be relieved of their duties, at least temporarily. often, it is the only legitimate means available to women.

ETHNIC DIFFERENCES

The difficulties of being old within an ethnic minority community also require separate consideration. It is generally assumed that ethnic minority elders live within supportive extended families, and that their need for professional care and support are invariably met within the family or cultural group.

Such stereotypical views oversimplify the diversity of ethnic groups, their distinctive cultures, religions, languages, individual life history, and the clashes that occur between the minority and dominant cultures. These can prevent access to services that might otherwise address their needs. The individual may have difficulty with English, or may be unfamiliar with indigenous social institutions. Moreover, institutional policies and practice have usually been developed in response to the specific needs of the indigenous population; many services are culture-bound, insensitive to different ways of life and beliefs. This is certainly true of what has been described as the 'ethnocentrism' of the NHS, and the 'colour blind' services provided by social work departments.

Recognition that ethnic minority elders face socially constructed dilemmas is increasing. Indeed, they run the risk of 'Triple Jeopardy' (Norman, 1985). The first is the discrimination which arises from ageing; in addition, older black people tend to suffer more socio-economic disadvantage relative to other groups. Thus, black elders share the marginalization and devaluation experienced by all older people. But an additional disadvantage arises from their cultural background, suffering discrimination because of their culture, religion, language and skin colour.

Loneliness and isolation is not an uncommon experience for ethnic elders. Even those supported within family and cultural groups may not receive the care and support that cultural norms demand. Isolation is relative, and can be associated with a level of family support that might be adequate for Western families, but falls short of cultural expectations. Loneliness can be a particular problem for Asian women, many of whom have never learnt English, and have spent most of their lives within the home. The losses they experience in old age can be particularly difficult to replace owing to the restricted nature of their social contacts.

Many Asian and Afro-Caribbean elders originally planned to return home, but were unable to do so. They now face ageing within social and family networks quite unlike those in indigenous communities, leading to particular stresses and disappointments which contribute to morbidity in old age. Many older people develop a particularly gloomy view of British life, believing that they can never be healthy here. They feel they have left behind factors associated with health: warmth, friendliness, fresh food and good company, and tend to associate Britain with illness, depression, worries, coldness, damp-ness, racism and loneliness (Donovan, 1986).

The discriminatory experience of ethnic minority groups also has an impact upon health. The racist idea that black people cause and spread disease has no basis in fact, although if there are statistics which apparently support such a belief, it is more likely rooted in the social conditions in which many black people live than in any racial characteristic. Given the disadvantages experienced by many older people from ethnic minorities, allied to our knowledge of the association between ill health and poverty, it should not be surprising that older black people tend to suffer poorer health than white people living in similar circumstances.

There are epidemiological differences between the various ethnic groups. Osteomalacia is common among older Asian women. Hypertension and stroke is more prevalent among Afro-Caribbeans, and ischaemic heart disease among Asians. The incidence of diabetes is higher among both Asian and Afro-Caribbeans than among the majority population (Fennel *et al.*, 1988; Whitehead *et al.*, 1988).

SEXUAL RELATIONSHIPS

Sex is an important element in human relationships, bringing pleasure, intimacy, personal fulfilment and self-esteem. Physical contact is a basic human need which probably becomes more important with ageing. Sexuality is an important means of communicating closeness and affection. Sexuality within relationships involves more than sexual intercourse. It involves companionship, friendship, the ability to relax intimately with another person, the pleasures of bodily contact through stroking, touching, caressing, and sharing cares and worries with another person.

The need, desire and capacity for sexual activity does not decline significantly with age; indeed, older people are as capable of loving passionately and tenderly as young people. Sexual relationships are spared the youthful pressures about 'performance', and can bring joy and tranquillity unknown in earlier years (Greengross and Greengross, 1989). Rather than ending sexual experience, age can extend the vocabulary of loving. Several studies have challenged the ageist belief that sexuality is an inevitable loss of old age, demonstrating that most older people continue to find sexual fulfilment and satisfaction (Kinsey's research of 1940s; Masters and Johnson, 1966; Hite, 1977). Older people continue to need the closeness and affirmation which sexual expression brings.

> Older adults are interested in sex, think about it, desire it, engage in it with the same frequency that Kinsey reported for forty year olds. Some 75% of respondents affirmed that sex was the same or better now than when younger.
> (Starr and Bakur-Weiner, 1982)

Yet whilst the physical and emotional value of sexual relationships is now recognized, there are many social, moral and religious beliefs which can deprive older people of the positive benefits of sexual relationships. They constitute an ageist denial of the sexuality of older people, leading to ideas which are misleading and damaging, implying that sex in old age is wrong, indecent, and even repellent. Many result from attitudes prevalent during formative years, which suggested that sexual activity for personal gratification, rather than childrearing, is sinful. As Comfort (1977) pointed out, this has a specific impact on older people, who can no longer use procreation as an 'excuse'.

Victorian and Edwardian social attitudes have exacerbated this problem. Distinct social and sexual roles were assigned to men and women. Many women expected little pleasure from sex, being taught that outside marrige it was sinful and dangerous, and that even when married sexual fulfilment should not be expected. Women were expected to be passive and submissive partners, excluded from sexual pleasure and repressing their sexual desires in order to maintain a ladylike' dignity. This was reinforced by the common belief that conception was deterred if women remained inactive and unaroused during intercourse.

The sexual liberation brought about by safer contraception, religious decline, and the major re-evaluation of women's social role, have led to these restrictive ideas being challenged. The idea that sex is for both male and female enjoyment has become common. However, this development is relatively recent, leaving many older people with considerable uncertainty. Many continue to accept the idea that sex for pleasure is sinful; others have changed their mind, many more are ambivalent, or embittered about lost opportunities.

Negative attitudes towards sexuality form part of ageism, and are held by people of all ages. Many younger people are reluctant to accept that older people, particularly parents, have any sexual desires or feelings. As Greengross and Greengross (1989) state, the impression given on television, films and advertising is that sex is only for the young and beautiful. Women, in particular, fear that ageing will result in them becoming sexually unattractive. Standards of beauty are concerned with the idealized pictures of youth, particularly the female 'pin-up', and it is unfortunate that those who do not conform to that single form of beauty are not identified with sexuality. Many older people accept that they are no longer considered attractive, and therefore cease to be sexual beings. But conventional visions of beauty should be widened from such restricted physical attributes. The beauty sought in people of all ages should be a reflection of inner warmth and energy, and an empathy towards other people.

Social ambivalence concerning the legitimate sexuality of older people produces serious personal problems. The ageist idea, shared by many professional carers, that sexuality is no longer a problem, and should not even be an issue in old age, can make it difficult for older people to obtain help and advice. The taboos restricting sexual activity do not alleviate human need for physical contact. Older generations have probably been subjected to more negative messages about sexual values and behaviour than any previous generation, and they remain powerful restraints on behaviour that can ultimately be unhealthy. The rejection of sexual relationships denies older people the health-giving benefits of the happiness, pleasure and enjoyment that they can bring.

In a multi-cutural society, moral views will vary. It is important that older people are not persuaded to participate in anything which offends them. Similarly, they should not be prevented, by religious or ageist dogma, from experiencing important aspects of sexual and personal relationships when they wish to do so. Yet even when released from powerful social and religious ideas, personal worries and uncertainties about sexuality have to be addressed. Many older people fear that ageing will bring about a decline in sexual excitement and pleasure. The sexual performance of men can be affected by fears of impotence; many women fear that the menopause will bring difficulties with vaginal lubrication, and painful intercourse. Such worries are largely unfounded; Masters and Johnson (1966) found that male fears were not age-related, with impotence and premature ejaculation being as applicable to younger as older men. They found that most problems are psychological rather than physical in origin. They also found that discomfort arising from vaginal lubrication was not a major problem in old age for 80% of women, and that even if it was, lubrication was possible.

For ageing people to continue to enjoy sexual activity, a positive attitude which determines to make the most of current capabilities, rather than regretting lost capacities, is helpful. Psychological problems are an important cause of difficulties. Many men have been brought up to associate maleness and virility with the ability to perform sex satisfactorily, and ageist fears about loss of power can itself lead to loss of performance.

Yet male sexuality can be influenced by other factors. Physical illness, such as diabetes or multiple sclerosis, Parkinson's disease and depression, can cause impotency, as can alcohol and nicotine. Many prescribed drugs affect sexual performance, such as those used to treat conditions like high blood pressure, both by reducing the ability to get or maintain an erection, and by preventing ejaculation. Some drugs can subdue all sexual feelings.

There are also social problems. Finding a new partner can be difficult, particularly for older women, who are more numerous and restrained by sexual mores, which allow older men to marry younger women, but not vice versa. Bereavement can often be worse when the survivor finds that he or she still has strong sexual feelings. Ageism often prevents older people turning to anyone for help, or seeking appropriate advice and reassurance, for fear that they will be ridiculed.

Even masturbation is difficult for many older people. The ancient Taoist religion thought that the process of ejaculation shortened life because it involved the loss of some important essence, or 'ching', with the seminal fluid. This belief has become widespread in many cultures, forming the basis for the belief that masturbation is weakening (Hunt, 1988). Many older people have been taught that masturbation is sinful, a potential hazard leading to mental illness, infertility and moral degeneration. This prevents many older people from utilizing this method of relief from sexual tension. Sex is a powerful instinct, and orgasm, shared or alone, is an important source of pleasure and contentment denied to many people (Greengross and Greengross, 1989).

The relationship between sex, health and old age is important. Many older people believe that sexual activity is unwise, that too much activity and excitement can damage health. The links between happiness and immunity to disease means that such ideas are almost certainly wrong. Even if correct, it might be better to die from living a full and active life, rather than dying from the frustration of restricting participation in enjoyable and necessary functions. Certainly, a happy, active and contented social life is probably the best antidepressant available; it is certainly one with the least side-effects.

Sexual activity provides excellent exercise when exercise is increasingly important to health. Moreover, the ability to maintain a sexual relationship is good reason for maintaining fitness and health, which both enables and encourages sexual activity. Indeed, the continuation of sexual activity into old age has been linked with increased longevity throughout history in many cultural groups (Georgakas, 1980).

Sexuality remains possible when older people suffer from chronic disease. After serious illness, when people need reassurance, the closeness of lying together, of feeling protected and cared for, may do more good than medical prescriptions. Often, in these private, intimate moments, couples can share their fears and anxieties, and reassure each other that they are still loved and valued. Two problems have to be overcome. The first relates to the dangers of heart attacks, brought on by excitement and over-exertion. Most modern medical advice would suggest that there is no need to eliminate sexual activity altogether unless heart disease is severe. Indeed, heart conditions may benefit from the moderate exercise of sexual activity, which can increase heart rate, normalize blood pressure, and improve oxygen consumption. Conversely, total sexual abstinence, arising from a rigid and fearful approach to life, can produce psychological stress which itself can aggravate heart disease.

The second problem concerns discomfort. The enjoyment of sex may be difficult if every movement causes pain, or if joints and limbs cannot be moved because of stiffness and discomfort. Arthritis can produce constant and nagging pain, making even the prospect of sexual activity so disagreeable that it can prevent arousal. The discomfort of sexual intercourse can be alleviated by a change of position; laying side-by-side can be more comfortable than the normal, 'missionary' position.

A POSITIVE ATTITUDE TO SOCIAL ENGAGEMENT

Older people need to dismiss the debilitating views which set limits on their ability to lead full and active lives. Old age is what we make it; it can be wretched, it can be abundant. Social involvement is a crucial element in old age. Older people need to develop a positive attitude to living, live adventurously, and challenge those aspects of ageism which suggest that older people should not do so. Good health is the basis for social involvement, but social involvement fosters good health. The individual needs to face the challenges which arise from full engagement in social life. Those who restrict their physical and mental involvement deteriorate both in body and mind. This decline can happen quickly, but more often it is insidiously slow, eroding our health over many years. The acceptance of personal challenges produces confidence, and it is confidence that makes it easier to meet fresh challenges.

7

Diet and nutrition

The idea that diet has a powerful impact on the maintenance of health can be traced to ancient times, with most older societies making no clear distinction between their pharmacopoeia and diet. Illich (1977) refers to a survey of German cookbooks which indicated that many were written by physicians who insisted that the best medicine comes from the kitchen rather than the pharmacy.

If drugs are defined as chemical compounds that seek a therapeutic effect upon the body, then food is indeed a drug. Modern nutrition is rediscovering the links between diet and health. Indeed, diet is probably the most important of all environmental factors affecting health. Food, after digestion, feeds the entire body, entering the blood stream and passing to every cell, supplying energy for movement, growth, and replenishing worn or damaged tissues.

Medicine recognizes the preventative importance of diet, but the main thrust of medical intervention continues to centre on complex surgical and drug treatment. Perhaps one reason is that effective dietary action can be undertaken simply by individuals, without the panoply of medical staff and technology normally involved in health care. In contrast, holistic approaches assume that every illness is traceable to internal disharmony, and whilst this can arise from many factors, the most common is nutritional.

There is firm evidence that nutrition plays an important role both in causing illness, and contributing to the ageing process.

Studies in experimental nutrition continue to correlate diet with immunity, disease, and longevity. The chronic diseases of the elderly are clearly related, to some degree, to dietary patterns, often established in early life and often changing or deteriorating in later life.

(Lamy, 1981)

The importance of nutrition can also be demonstrated by national and cultural comparisons. For instance, the Japanese, who tend to have a longer life expectancy than people from Western nations, eat simple food, prepared from fresh, natural ingredients. The diseases of 'Western' culture, including constipation, obesity, diverticular disease, diabetes, coronary heart disease, and colon cancer, which plague the lives of many older people, are virtually unknown by those who have kept to traditional Japanese cuisine. They are, however, becoming more common with those who have adopted Western eating habits.

So changing national diet patterns can improve the state of national health. It is widely accepted that the average British diet is closely linked to modern Western disease. Moreover, preventative dietary changes are general rather than disease specific, indicating that improved nutrition will help prevent most, if not all disease.

During most of human evolution, mankind were basically hunter-gatherers, their workload light, infant mortality high, and with little or no malnutrition, although people probably ate fewer calories than desired (Schauss, 1985). Only comparatively recently has human diet changed fundamentally; indeed, there are strong indications that modern diet has become so far removed from natural requirements that the body is now failing to adjust, with digestion, absorption, assimilation, utilization and elimination all functioning under stress, with lowered overall efficiency. Increased susceptibility to illness is the result.

The main difference between 'traditional' and 'modern' eating patterns concern developments in food technology. It is not an exaggeration to suggest that food processing has made British diet positively lethal. Schauss (1985) has outlined the main changes. Since 1800, the consumption of dietary bulk and roughage has dropped sharply as refined carbohydrate (principally sugar and flour) has increased. The consumption of salt and fat has also increased, and since the 1920s hydrogenated oil has been in use. More recently, convenience foods have appeared, and artificial food additives have been successfully combined to produce foods that have become widely distributed and consumed.

Older generations were first subjected to the early promotion of the 'new' foods, high in fat, low in dietary fibre, with higher sugar and salt contents. Processed white bread replaced bread made from the wholegrain. Tinned fruit and vegetables replaced fresh supplies. Sugar sweetened the appetite for a multitude of appealing new products. The health consequences have been devastating. Food is now so refined, processed and adulterated with chemicals that many believe that the industrialized production of food is the key to modern disease.

The influence of the food processing industry, which continues to produce food on the basis of profitability rather than health, is immense. This is supported by government policies which do little to provide incentives for a healthier diet. People rely increasingly on convenience and processed foods, not least older people who find that they are quicker, easier and cheaper to buy, prepare, cook and eat. Poverty is another factor which often affects the ability of older people to change their diet.

Modern food production creates health problems through toxicology or poisoning, and allergy. Long-standing fears concerning the effects of chemical additives and contaminants in food, crop spraying, and the impact of artificial fertilizers on the soil are beginning to be realized. The mass production of meat has produced two major problems: infection and behaviour disorders. Poultry, for instance, are reared in overcrowded indoor conditions, devoid of sun or contact with the soil, and are fed on processed foods containing pesticides and hormones. The recent outbreak of 'mad-cow disease' has been explained, at least in part, by the feeding of meat pellets to animals that are entirely vegetarian. The result is unhealthy animals, treated with antibiotics, fungicides and tranquillizers, all degrading the food they become by leaving chemical residues which are now recognized to be an increasing threat to human health.

A large number of compounds never before ingested by humans or other animals became common in the diet, with almost completely unknown and poorly monitored consequences for hepatic, neuroendocrine, cardiovascular, and immunological biochemistry, and particularly for fetal developmental biochemistry and biochemical genetics.

(Schauss, 1985)

There are a number of specific problems which have consequences on human health, particularly for older people. The over-consumption of fat provides more calories than people require, often resulting in obesity. Fat consumption increases the risk of many forms of cancer, heart disease, high blood pressure, diabetes and arthritis. Many digestive problems, from constipation to diverticular disease, are linked with fat consumption. There is also some evidence that saturated fat leads to premature ageing (Straten, 1987). The consumption of meat, cream, eggs, cream cheese and hard cheese, butter, lard, margarine, and other foods made from animal fat, needs to be drastically reduced.

The consumption of refined carbohydrates, particularly sugar, has also risen enormously. Sugar is a highly concentrated form of energy, providing abundant calories, but almost no nourishment. Simple scientific tests indicate why the body cannot cope with large influxes of sugar.

Put proteins in a concentrated solution of sugar and you can watch the transformation. The sugar slowly binds to the proteins, permanently altering their molecular structure and . . . the way they work. It now seems that we too go yellowy-brown on standing – on ageing, that is. It happens as excess sugar in the diet attacks proteins in our bodies.

(Furth and Harding, 1989)

Many diseases, such as coronary heart disease and diabetes, are now associated with sugar consumption. It is certainly implicated in the modern epidemic of hypoglycaemia, recognized by irrational behaviour, emotional instability, distorted judgement, and unpleasant personality defects. These include sensitivity to criticism, irritability and hostile behaviour, insomnia, sleep disturbances, restlessness, night terrors, chronic fatigue, depression, recurrent fevers of unknown origin, abdominal and chest pains, and headaches (Schauss, 1985). Hypoglycaemia is also the result of eating habits. Many people start the day with coffee, a sweet breakfast cereal, followed by a cigarette. Anyone who eats pure sugar on an empty stomach will find that the levels of blood glucose shoot up and, with ageing, the more pronounced and prolonged the rise in blood glucose can become. The combination of caffeine, sugar and nicotine triggers a flood of insulin into the system causing blood glucose to fall below normal levels. (Cheraskin *et al.*, 1974).

Diabetics, who have raised levels of glucose in the blood, are significantly more prone to cataracts, and more likely to suffer from atherosclerosis, the clogging of arteries. This also causes damage to the kidneys and circulation (Furth and Harding, 1989).

The importance of dietary fibre, or roughage, has been rediscovered in recent years. Fibre comes from the cell walls of plants such as wheat, rice, fruit, vegetables, pulses and nuts, in two distinct varieties, both essential to health. Pectin, found in apples and grapes is a potent cholesterol-lowering agent. Cellulose, found in nuts and cereals, assists in the formation of stool bulk.

Late nineteenth-century milling methods were able to remove bran, the fibre-rich husk of the wheat, and the wheatgerm, the tiny embryo wheatplant rich in nutrients. This has resulted in white bread containing little fibre and few vitamins. During the same period, eating habits reduced the consumption of fruit, vegetables, pulses and nuts in favour of animal fats. Meat, eggs and dairy products contain no fibre, and sweetened refined foods further reduce the consumption of fibre-rich food.

Fibre deficiency is linked to various illnesses, including haemorrhoids, diverticulosis, diabetes, heart disease and cancer. By lowering blood cholesterol, fibre inhibits the development of arteriosclerotic heart disease. Constipation is a common complaint which is assisted by increasing dietary fibre. Allied with regular exercise, it is a condition that can be cured without resort to medication. Eating rich, spicy food, especially meat, is now associated with cancer of the intestines and bowels, for without fibrous material encouraging defecation, cancer can ensue from putrefying food passing more slowly through the intestine, forming poisonous, carcinogenic waste products.

The modern diet of refined and processed foods is now also contaminated by chemical substances which act as stabilizers, flavourants, extenders, colours, preservatives and antioxidants, all added to improve the keeping qualities, taste, texture and colour of manufactured foods and drinks during storage, handling, transportation, freezing and reheating. There has not been time for extensive study of their long-term effects on health, but most evidence suggests they are harmful. They are being identified as a hazard to food-allergic consumers, incriminated as causative agents in a wide range of behavioural problems and learning disorders, as well as asthma, hyperactivity, urticaria, digestive disturbances and other allergic illness (Mackarness, 1980).

THE DIETARY NEEDS OF OLDER PEOPLE

The popular idea that dietary needs diminish with ageing should be challenged. The available evidence suggests that nutrient requirements do not vary significantly with age, except perhaps for a slight reduction in the need for calories, although even this might result from reduced physical activity, which is not to be recommended.

However, older people do experience a range of factors that make it appear that they have a diminishing need for food. These increase the risk of nutritional deficiency. Some are physical, such as the loss of teeth, the decline of taste and smell, immobility and poor vision. Some are emotional, such as loneliness, bereavement, apathy and depression, all known to suppress appetite. Some concern chronic illness, such as arthritis, many infections, stomach disorders and cancer. Others are structural, for example, low income, the absence of social companionship (eating is a social as well as a health-related habit), and immobility related to the effort required to purchase and prepare food.

Older people require a comprehensive intake of all nutrients, particularly protein, calcium, iron, potassium, ascorbic acid and vitamin D. An inadequate or unbalanced diet is more harmful for older people. Foods tolerated in earlier years of more robust health can become dangerous to older people, leading to specific health deficits. Many features of chronic ailments associated with ageing, such as anaemia, behavioural and neurological deterioration, connective tissue changes and muscle weakness, are also early signs of dietary deficiency. What is becoming clear is that such symptoms are not necessarily the unavoidable features of ageing, but the result of inadequate diet.

There is a common assumption that illness caused by malnutrition no longer occurs in this country. The consistent message from the Ministry of Agriculture, Fisheries and Food in its quarterly *National Food Survey*, is that there is ongoing progress towards a healthier diet. Such evidence can be challenged. Government surveys in 1972 and 1979 found that malnutrition amongst older people lingers, but perhaps more important, there exists a level of 'subclinical' malnutrition, particularly of energy, iron, thiamine, folate, ascorbic acid, and vitamin D, all crucial elements in health maintenance.

The association between old age and poverty is probably the most important determinant of inadequate nutrition amongst older people. *National Food Surveys* show clear links between family income and consumption of essential nutrients, and low-income families are less likely to be able to make changes towards the currently recommended 'healthy' diets (British Social Attitudes, 1987). The basic pension does not encourage older people to purchase an adequate diet, creating instead a reliance upon cheaper, processed foods.

Prolonged malnutrition speeds the ageing process, leading to weakness, listlessness, and apathy. These factors, so often associated with old age rather than diet, can often result from, and in, a lack of energy (Cheraskin *et al.*, 1974). Many illnesses of old age, often caused by poor nutrition, have an impact on the desire for food, creating another classic vicious circle. These problems, which constrain the capacity for dietary change, need to be addressed when encouraging people to adopt healthier nutrition.

Yet malnutrition does not necessarily emanate from lack of food; overweight people are not necessarily well nourished, and can often be deficient in protein, fibre, vitamins and minerals. Consuming starchy foods, sweet foods and sugared drinks can all increase weight without nutritional benefit.

Obesity is a health hazard for many older people. It can arise from restricted physical activity, which reduces food requirements, with excess consumption being deposited as fatty tissue. Eating can also provide comfort to people who are worried, bored or depressed. Once overweight, fat can become difficult to lose, particularly when an individual feels unattractive, and there appears to be little point in doing so.

Overweight people are more prone to heart disease, high blood pressure, hypertension, atherosclerosis, varicose veins, diabetes and arthritis, and obesity is an added danger in surgery and recovery from operations. Even mild obesity is unhealthy. Additional weight places added strain on the heart, joints, spine and legs. This in turn can reduce mobility, establishing a vicious circle of more weight, less mobility, too much food, and increased weight (Cheraskin *et al.*, 1974).

The consumption of alcohol, tea and coffee can also become a problem, particularly considering the large quantities consumed by many older people. Caffeine, nicotine and alcohol are legalized drugs, which can cause more damage to both mind and body than all proscribed and prescribed drugs combined. Caffeine is found in coffee, tea, cola drinks, cocoa and chocolate, limited amounts of which contain sufficient to stimulate the brain, sharpen the senses, distort muscular co-ordination, and hamper timing. Caffeine stimulates insulin secretion, causing blood-sugar levels to drop, which can cause a hypoglycaemic condition (Cheraskin *et al.*, 1974). Tannin in tea and coffee can reduce iron absorbtion from 20–60% when consumed with meals (Schauss, 1985).

Excessive alcohol can cause malnutrition, premature ageing and weight problems. It is often assumed that malnutrition is the result of alcoholism rather than a contributing factor, but the malnutrition of brain cells has been found to cause alcoholism (Cheraskin *et al.*, 1974).

The association between tea and coffee drinking with addiction, may appear an over-reaction, but all three beverages display the three signs characteristic of addiction: tolerance for the drug, withdrawal symptoms when it is removed, and craving for it after deprivation. The withdrawal symptoms of heavy coffee drinkers include headaches, irritability, nervousness, restlessness, inability to work and lethargy. Another coffee can promptly relieve the symptoms.

Smoking has also been found to create a desire for caffeine and sugar. Smokers drink more coffee, heavily sugared, than non-smokers (Cheraskin *et al.*, 1974).

Perhaps herbal teas can be recommended to replace them. These are beneficial to health, and much enjoyment can be gained by sampling new teas. Phillips (1983) outlines the values of some teas, for example, dandelion detoxifies the liver; dill aids sleep; jasmine calms the nerves; nettle assists low blood pressure; and comfrey is highly recommended for its healing properties. Ceres (1984) mentions many others which promote relaxation, sleep and cheerfulness, all without the danger of habit-forming dependency.

FOOD ALLERGIES AND INTOLERANCE

Although allergic illnesses have been described since ancient times, they are still imperfectly understood. Allergy means an unusual or altered response to contact with a substance foreign to the body (Mackarness, 1980). Allergies are commonly associated with sneezing and tearful eyes; but there are allergic reactions which affect the heart, stomach, bowels, skin, the nervous system, and, indeed, can disrupt every major physiological system within the body (Watson, 1972).

Chemical allergy can arise from the use of sprays, polishes, natural gas and oil, central heating, prescribed drugs and many other aspects of the physical environment. Foods are chemicals, and food allergy cannot be easily separated from chemical allergy, particularly as so much food now contains chemical contaminants (Mackarness, 1980). Food allergy is the reaction experienced immediately after the consumption of a particular food, ranging from a runny nose to total physical collapse.

Food intolerance, in contrast, occurs over a longer period, with more varied consequences. The delayed reaction of food intolerance, combined with the fact that the offending food is often part of staple diet, can prevent direct connections between food and illness being made. The orthodox medical view of food intolerance is sceptical. It is, indeed, hard to imagine that some common foods, such as wheat, milk and eggs, eaten regularly by large numbers of people, can cause migraine, headaches, painful joints, diarrhoea, hyperactivity, fatigue, asthma and eczema in some people. A large proportion of food intolerance concern individuals who crave the very foods that cause their physical or mental symptoms. The continual eating of a food to which an allergy has developed can keep the patient feeling good for many years, so long as that food is taken frequently. Omission will produce withdrawal or hangover symptoms, relieved by resorting to more of the same food (Mackarness, 1980).

Allergy and intolerance are individualized complaints. The symptoms that develop, and how bad they are, will depend on the individual. There is no single diet suitable for everyone. The general rule is to follow the principles of good diet, but thereafter allergy and intolerance become a personal matter. There is, however, more chance of a reaction if the individual is unwell, or engaged in emotional conflict (Mackarness, 1976).

DIET AND MENTAL HEALTH

Nutritional deficiency can cause mental illness. In recent years, researchers have examined many psychological conditions and found evidence which suggests that considerable emotional distress is caused, or worsened, by nutritional imbalance. This should not be surprising. Food provides nutrients which the bloodstream carries to the brain, so any interference with nutritional supply can result in impaired functioning. Food intolerance affects all aspects of the body, so the brain, the most sensitive part of the body, will almost certainly suffer allergic reactions to foods or other chemicals that surround us. Indeed, if deprived of essential proteins, vitamins, and minerals, brain cells degenerate rapidly, and a deteriorating emotional and intellectual state can result (Cheraskin *et al.*, 1974).

Behavioural conditions can result from poor nutrition. Many links between diet, feelings and behaviour have focused on young people. Although many of the more serious links probably remain unproven, it is suspected that much deviant child behaviour can arise from nutrient deficiencies, leading to increased impulsiveness, a reduction in inhibitory control, and a reduction in the fear of social consequences (Schauss, 1985). Similar problems almost certainly affect older people, even though evidence is not as readily available.

Food can also act positively. Studies have indicated that when people eat carbohydrates their mood immediately becomes more relaxed and calm. Wurtman (1988) explains how carbohydrates apparently trigger a calming chemical in the brain, which causes negative feelings to die down and anger to vanish. Yet other evidence

(Watson, 1976; Cheraskin *et al.*, 1974; Mackarness, 1980; Schauss, 1985) indicates that even foods commonly considered to be wholesome and good, such as milk and eggs, may adversely affect older people.

> Some neurological diseases have been attributed to folic acid deficiency because some patients with such disorders, most of whom were elderly, have responded to folic acid supplements. Deficiencies of other nutrients, such as tryptophan and thiamine, have also been suggested as causes for behaviour changes in the elderly. It has also been found that multivitamin supplements have decreased morbidity in elderly long-stay patients.
>
> (Schorah and Morgan, 1985)

There are suggestions that confusion might have a dietary element. Lamy (1981) predicted that increased attention to nutritional factors in health and disease may eventually enable the use of diet to prevent or reverse the damage done to the brain by Alzheimer's disease or related problems. Asplund *et al.*, (1981) noted that Alzheimer patients have low blood glucose levels, and that diabetes is notably uncommon, quoting research which indicated links between dietary status and mental decline. Runcie (1981) found that vitamin B deficiency characteristically gives rise to confusion, and that long-standing folate deficiency also causes a confusional state. The links between malnutrition and chronic psychic disorders is an area of research that should be pursued in order to assist the task of looking after the increasing number of elderly, mentally infirm people.

A DIET FOR GOOD HEALTH IN OLD AGE

Sensible eating habits promote good health. It is not intended to detail what constitutes good diet here, as many books are available which deal with the subject. Instead, the general recommendations taken by holistic approaches to health will be outlined. These are important in extending health into old age, and the task of preventing and overcoming the illnesses which reduce the quality of life older people can expect.

Proper nutrition has to supply all the substances necessary for maintaining health, strength and energy, without causing overweight. The type of food eaten, and how much, are important factors which can safeguard against the four main hazards of incorrect nutrition: obesity, malnutrition, inadequate nutrition, and increased risk of diet-related disease. Good diet also maintains the immune system, ensures protection from disease, and a feeling of health, enthusiasm and confidence upon which older people can base an active and continuing social involvement.

The principles of improved diet are now well understood, and they are particularly relevant to the health of older people. The general principles are to:

1. Reduce fat consumption: the number of people suffering from heart disease and cancer has been closely linked with the amount of fat and animal products consumed, primarily meat, milk, butter and cheese.
2. Reduce the consumption of refined carbohydrates, principally sugar: sugar is an 'empty calorie' food, which produces energy, but no other useful nutrient.
3. Increase the consumption of fibre: dietary fibre is not digested by the body, but is helpful in its assistance in passing food quickly through the body, and providing bulk to make stools solid.
4. Avoid foods containing additives: these have been added to food to make them look better and keep longer. They play no part in maintaining health, and many can directly damage health. This advice includes the use of salt, which is now implicated in hypertension, and all related heart disease. Older people can be particularly sensitive to this.

Guidelines for healthy eating centre upon a balanced and varied diet, made up chiefly of fresh wholefoods, particularly vegetables and fruit, wholemeal bread, rice, potatoes and pasta. This involves eating less refined and processed food containing sugar, salt and additives, less meat, butter, full-fat milk, less fried food, cakes, sweets; less tea, coffee and alcohol. With these provisos, a varied diet is important, not least as the taste, flavour and aroma of different foods stimulates the secretion of digestive juices, which are themselves responsible for the correct transformation and utilization of food. This makes it sensible to avoid routine eating patterns often witnessed with older people.

Unfortunately, many factors now known to constitute good diet will have to be 'unlearnt'. It became fashionable for older generations to eat white bread; meat was not only healthy, but displayed affluence; refined foods have been presented as attractive and wholesome; and sugar was considered to be white, sweet and pure. The dietary restrictions of the Second World War enhanced such feelings. People wanted what was not available, even though the wartime diet was probably healthier than the diet of post-war affluence.

Improving diet will often mean decreased consumption of foods that many people love, and returning to foods that older people have spent a lifetime being persuaded to abandon. Hence it is not an easy task, however important it is to the maintenance of health.

The problem with animal products, particularly meat, eggs and dairy produce, is their high-fat and cholesterol content. People with high levels of cholesterol in their blood run increased risks of heart disease and cancer in later life. Cholesterol is produced within the body, and does not require additional dietary sources, and the last 100 years has seen an unprecedented rise in the consumption of cholesterol-rich food.

Special diets have been developed to prevent and cure particular ailments, and these can be effective with many conditions which medicine considers to be 'incurable'. Thorsons, the publishers, have brought out a series of booklets entitled, *Diets to Help* . . . , covering such matters as arthritis, bronchial troubles, constipation, diabetes, hypertension, prostate troubles, heart disorders and many others. The validity of the dietary claims made in such texts is being confirmed by an increasing number of people who can personally testify to their effectiveness.

Dietary vitamins and minerals are essential for older people, as they are involved in all biochemical reactions within the body. Vitamins are necessary for the well-being of cells, tissues and organs, and for the metabolic balance of the whole organism. Their value probably increases with age, and whilst a balanced diet should supply adequate quantities, several studies have found that the diets of older people are often deficient, resulting in ailments generally associated with old age (Schorah and Morgan, 1985). Some studies have indicated that many conditions associated with ageing may be no more than vitamin deficiencies, particularly of vitamin D.

Serious deficits can lead to deficiency diseases, such as scurvy, pernicious anaemia, pellagra, beri-beri, and rickets. Schorah and Morgan (1985) found that about 1% of ageing people in industrialized areas have scurvy, usually amongst older people who eat insufficient fresh vegetables and fruit.

Small deficits are more usual, and less often detected, but over a number of years, these can adversely affect bodily functioning, impairing the efficiency of the immune process, and lead to illness. Brain cells are particularly vulnerable, and any shortage will alter brain function. Many nutrients are not manufactured within the body, but are acquired through diet, either coming from the gut after digestion, or synthesized and secreted from various organs, including the liver. When this process is impeded, problems can arise that affect health.

Although less work has been done with dietary deficiency in older people, potential links can be deduced from the following summary of the effects such deficiency. This information, gathered from a number of sources, is intended as a guide to discern whether specific illnesses, contracted by specific individuals, could have a nutritional basis.

ESSENTIAL VITAMINS AND MINERALS

Vitamins and minerals are part of the structure of every cell in the body, and are fundamentally important to the maintenance of health, particularly in the later years of life.

Vitamin A (retinol) This is associated with resistance to infections, healthy mucous membranes, the prevention of anaemia, skin conditions, night vision and permanent blindness. It is widely distributed in green vegetables, carrots, fish, eggs, milk, butter and cheese.

B complex vitamins These are vital in preventing anaemia, and maintaining healthy nerves and muscular energy. They are all water soluble, and are easily lost in the process of cooking, freezing and preserving. Alcohol, smoking, drugs and stress can all prevent the body absorbing them efficiently, particularly in old age.

Vitamin B_1 (thiamine) This is sometimes called 'the morale vitamin' because of its positive effects on the nervous system. When absent from the diet, reserves in body tissue are drawn upon, including tissue from the brain and central nervous system, eventually compromising brain function. Deficiency is associated with loss of appetite, bowel disorders, depressions, irritability, confusion, memory loss, lack of concentration, loss of co-ordination and sensitivity to noise. Deficiency can be caused by excessive alcohol intake and can lead to cardiac failure. It is not stored in the body, but is widely available in most vegetables and fruit, nuts, seafood, meat, especially hearts and liver, whole grains and rice.

Vitamin B_2 (riboflavin) This is associated with the growth and repair of body tissue and the health of red blood cells. Deficiency can lead to depression, learning difficulties, insomnia, lack of energy, skin conditions and degenerating eyesight. It is widely distributed in all foods including dairy produce, seeds and nuts, liver, yeast, milk, eggs, green vegetables and fruit.

Vitamin B_3 (niacin)   This is required for digestion, hormone production, regulating blood pressure and cholesterol levels, and its absence is associated with nervous and mental disorders, including insomnia, exhaustion, irritability, confusion, dementia, depression and hallucination, as well as stomach upsets and skin disorders. It is available in beans and peas, wholegrain cereals, eggs, fish, liver, lean meats, vegetables and fruit.

Vitamin B_5 (pantothenic acid)   This is the antistress vitamin, valuable in avoiding depression. It also produces antibodies which fight infection, and aids many metabolic functions. Its absence can lead to fatigue, sleep disturbance, nausea, digestive problems, impaired co-ordination, depression and inability to tolerate stress. It is widely distributed in food, especially whole grains, yeast, eggs, nuts, liver, milk and broccoli.

Vitamin B_6 (pyridoxine)   This is involved in the utilization of proteins, and is associated with irritability, convulsions, muscular twitching, dermatitis near the eyes, neuritis and kidney stones. It is available in yeast, liver, lean meat and wholegrain cereals.

Vitamin B_{12} (cyanocobalamine)   This is required in every cell, particularly red blood cells, muscle, nerves and the intestines. It helps to utilize iron, prevents anaemia, assists in the maintenance of the bone marrow, gives energy, and maintains nervous health. Its absence can lead to difficulty in concentration and memory, tiredness, irritability, depression, hallucinations, manic or paranoid behaviour, anaemia, and neurological disorders. It is available in dairy products, yoghurt, lean meat, liver, fish and eggs.

Vitamin C (ascorbic acid)   This is required for the production of connective tissues, the fighting of infection, the healing of wounds, brain and nerve function, the formation of bones, the strength and health of blood vessels, and various digestive functions. Vitamin C also increases resistance to infections. It is not produced or stored within the body, so is dependent on dietary sources. Deficiency is commonly asssociated with scurvy, the degeneration of skin, teeth and blood vessels, but can also lead to anaemia, irritability, muscle pain, joint swelling, delayed wound healing, including pressure areas and varicose ulcers, and lead to an increased risk of atherosclerosis and other heart disease. It is available mainly in citrus fruits, blackcurrants, blackberries and rosehips, but is also present in most vegetables, notably tomatoes, although it is easily destroyed in preparation and cooking.

Vitamin D   This is the sunshine vitamin, synthesized in the skin under the influence of sunlight. It regulates the absorbtion of calcium and phosphorus supplies within the body, and so it is essential for strong bones and teeth, and for combatting osteomalacia in older people. It is available from margarine, eggs, dairy products, and fatty fish, such as herrings, tuna, sardines, salmon and cod-liver oil.

Vitamin E (tocopherol)   This functions to promote normal blood clotting, detoxifies pollutants within the body, helps to regenerate the skin, controls cholesterol levels, protects against the decalcification of bones, joints and soft tissue, and acts as an antioxidant to prevent cell membrane damage. Deficiency can lead to irritability, fatigue, muscle weakness and cramp. There is some evidence that it is effective in combatting multiple sclerosis. It is available from seeds, rice, green leafy vegetables, avocado, soya, sesame and vegetable oils, and margarine.

Vitamin H (biotin)   This is important for the production of proteins and fats, and the oxidation of carbohydrates and fatty acids. Deficiency can cause increased cholesterol levels, fatigue, depression, lassitude, insomnia, panic, hallucinations, nausea, dermatitis and muscular pains. It is available in legumes, vegetables and meats.

Vitamin K (phylloquinone)   This is important in blood clotting, and is associated with severe bleeding and internal haemorrhages, and can help to avoid strokes. It is also important in liver function. It is available from green vegetables, cauliflowers, milk, eggs and polyunsaturated oils.

Vitamin M (folic acid)   This is required for the production of blood cells, the breakdown and utilization of proteins, and for iron within the body. Deficiency can cause anaemia, insomnia, gastrointestinal disturbances, irritability, mental impairment, nerve degeneration, and neurological diseases. It is available in beans and peas, green leafy vegetables, liver, eggs, fish, yeast, green vegetables and wholegrain products.

Calcium   This is an essential mineral for the bones and teeth, and is often lacking in the diet of older people. It is also essential for normal blood clotting, the elasticity of connective tissue, the immune system, the blood supply and the nervous system. Its absence can cause anxiety, fatigue, depression, insomnia, muscle cramp and, in older people, osteoporosis. It is available in milk, cheese, yoghurt, nuts and green vegetables.

Iron   This is part of haemoglobin, which is responsible for transporting oxygen in blood. It is necessary for preventing anaemia and resisting disease. Low iron levels cause tiredness, lethargy, headaches, breathlessness and loss of appetite. It can also impair judgement, reasoning, weaken inhibitory control, and damage intellectual and verbal skills. Iron is available in eggs, lean meats, whole grains, liver, bread, potatoes, green vegetables, apricots and cherries.

Magnesium   This is stored in the bones, and is vital for nerve conduction, muscular contraction, and the transmission of impulses along the nervous system. Deficiency can cause weakness, insomnia, heart disorders, convulsions, hallucinations, confusion and disorientation. It is available in apples, bananas, fish, nuts, seeds, peas, beans, wholegrains and green vegetables.

Phosphorus   This is part of every cell and chemical reaction in the body, and is found particularly in the bones and teeth. It is required for the muscles, good eyesight, and the metabolism of food. Deficiencies can lead to weakness, irritability, nervousness, loss of weight, heart disorders, and mental disorientaiton. It is available in milk, cheese, meat, beans, peas and grains.

Potassium   This is an important constituent of nervous tissue, essential for the brain, nerve function and body/water balance. Its absence is associated with muscular weakness and mental confusion, but also respiratory failure, irregular heartbeat, constipation, fatigue and insomnia. It is available in nuts, wholegrains, milk, fruit and green vegetables.

Selenium   This is an essential trace element, now much scarcer owing to farming methods which have removed it from the soil. Its absence is known to produce accelerated ageing, low resistance to infection, and wasting diseases, and so is particularly important to the maintenance of health in ageing. It is available in fish, garlic, onions, liver, tuna, eggs, brown rice, asparagus and bran.

Zinc   This is essential to many body functions, with deficiency causing apathy, poor appetite, loss of taste and smell, hair loss, and decreased immunity from infection. Food processing and zinc-depleted soils produce plants, fruits, vegetables, grains and animals in which zinc is absent. Otherwise, it is available in sea food, such as herring, oysters, sardines, brown rice, nuts, seeds, eggs and dairy produce.

There are other minerals, trace elements, which are needed in minute quantities, and without which the body cannot function properly, including cobalt, copper, iodine, manganese, selenium and molybdenum.

Some nutritional deficiencies are iatrogenic. Lamy (1981) claimed that food-drug interactions are probably more common than are generally believed. Posner (1979) outlined numerous examples of adverse drug-diet interactions; folate deficiency can be produced by anticonvulsants; antibiotics can produce vitamin deficiency. Chronic use or abuse of medications can produce gastrointestinal abnormalities, which affect nutritional status. Potassium deficiency can be caused by laxatives, which can also create mental confusion and depression.

To counteract vitamin and mineral deficiency, daily supplements are often recommended. However, it should be realized that whilst excess doses of many vitamins are harmless, large doses of vitamin A and vitamin D may be harmful.

THE BENEFITS OF FASTING AND UNDERNUTRITION.

Many medical writers, from Aristotle to Avicenna, have taught that dietary restriction enhances health, with more recent evidence confirming that illness and disease can be caused as much by excessive diet, or eating too much of the wrong things, as malnutrition. Exton-Smith (1971) concluded that overfeeding after maturity increases the incidence of degenerative diseases in later life. The major dietary problem is perhaps no longer lack of food, or even poverty, but excessive nutrition.

The idea that restricted diet can lead to longer life is based on work done with experimental animals (Fulder, 1983; Hunt, 1988), the conclusion being that it might add between 40 and 80 years to human lifespan. The research not only emphasized the life-extending properties of restricted diet, but also the delayed onset of age-related diseases, such as arthritis, cancer, heart and kidney disease. It can also affect susceptibility to disease, physiological performance, mental alertness and intelligence. Cancers, cataracts, discoloration and matting of hair, dryness of skin, kidney disease, and heart disease, have all been found to be less frequent in animals with restricted, rather than normal diets. Those animals that developed disease did so at a substantially later age than their unrestricted partners.

Walford (1983) is a major proponent of undernutrition (as opposed to malnutriton or inadequate nutrition), where the total intake of calories is gradually limited without reducing the critical nutrients vital to health. He believes that undernutrition works by protecting the body's immune system from the wear and tear of normal ageing, enabling it to continue functioning further into old age.

The health advantage of dietary control and fasting has always been a feature of some alternative medical advice. The benefits claimed vary from restoring appetite, bringing back vigour, virility and fertility, sharpening senses, including memory, brightening the skin, and clearing the eyes. Fasting has been likened to house-cleaning (Phillips, 1983), allowing a slow, natural cleansing of the body. When allied with total rest, fasting enables the body to regain its vigour and health.

The value of fasting has to be understood in relation to the energy used by the body in digesting food. Digestion breaks down food into its component nutrients, building these into cellular tissue, or using them for energy. The residue is then ejected from the body through the usual eliminative organs, the kidney, the bowels, the lungs and the skin. Even when the body is dealing with the smallest quantity of food, this process of assimilation is dominant. If too much food, or food containing considerable quantities of unwanted toxic matter, is regularly ingested, the body will not deal adequately with the build-up of toxins and waste matter. These accumulate within the body, ultimately causing illness and disease. Fasting allows the body to cleanse itself, directing its energy into elimination, and the maintenance of other body functions.

Conventional advice for older people is that they require regular meals, and that fasting might be injurious to health. This underestimates the ability of the body to live on its energy reserves. Whilst chronological age and personal health clearly have to be taken into consideration, as does the nature and duration of the fast, the value of fasting for older people should not be dismissed. Certainly, the reduction of diet must not be embarked upon too sharply; a gradual restriction of calories has been found to be the key to effectiveness, achieved by a general daily reduction, or by fasting completely for one or two days per week.

The limit of fasting for older, sick people occurs only when disease is at an advanced stage, or where the body has no further reserves of energy to deal with the condition. Starvation commences only after these reserves have been exhausted, after which fasting will lead to the break-down of muscle tissue and organs, and eventually lead to death. Despite the caution necessary, Phillips (1983) suggests that after certain major illnessess, such as a stroke, the only effective solution is a fast.

Indeed, the benefits of fasting are most likely to apply to older people, for they have suffered the longest build-up of toxicity. This is an alternative explanation for older people suffering from wasting diseases; not simply the result of ageing, but the toxic build-up that malnutrition and overnutrition creates over a lifetime.

To the extent that nutrition can determine our personal health, there are two important lessons that can be learnt. First, the maintenance of health becomes more clearly under individual control than most people currently believe. It certainly removes it from being the exclusive preserve of the medical profession, its pills, science and technology. Second, it challenges the dominant ageist assumptions which attribute the physical and mental illnesses of older people to the inevitable and irreversible process of ageing.

Furthermore, carers of older people should begin to examine the links between good health in old age and nutrition. New health and social work tasks become evident, both through advising older people about their diet, and through the nutritional content of meals supplied directly via hospital canteens, 'meals on wheels', and day and residential care units for older people. All available evidence suggests that good diet maintains health and can lead to an improved quality of life for older people. Many health and social work clients rely on the food provided for them, and so instead of seeing this as the provision of a practical service, meals should be seen as central to a wider strategy aimed at maintaining the health of older people.

It is often difficult to change the eating preferences of older people who feel that even proven nutritional hazards have hitherto caused them no harm. However, this fails to recognize the older body is less able to withstand bad eating habits with the immunity enjoyed by younger people. Although it is widely believed that changed diet would be effective only if started earlier in life, dietary restriction studies have indicated that considerable advantages to both lifespan and health can accrue even when dietary change is begun in midadulthood, or later.

8

Physical aspects of health: exercise, posture and relaxation

The value of exercise has been known since the days of ancient Greece, when recreational and competitive sports were pursued in the understanding that a fit individual was synonymous with a healthy individual (Ashton and Davies, 1986). However, since the Industrial Revolution, links between health and exercise have gradually diminished. Modern technology at work, within the home, and for transportation, has made it possible to live comfortably with a minimum of physical effort. Physical exercise, once a necessity, has become a matter of choice, with the result that life in modern society, more than at any previous time, has become sedentary and inactive.

This is particularly so for older people, who have increasingly been expected to rest and relax for their own good. The implication is that health can be harmed, indeed, life placed at risk, if older people exert themselves too strenuously. The 'rate of living' theory originated from late nineteenth-century ideas which suggested that the more energy expended, and the more oxygen dissipated, the shorter lifespan becomes. These ideas were based on an analogy between machines and the human body, and were particularly pernicious to older people. Machines wear out with use, and when the body is viewed as a machine, they too can be expected to deteriorate the more they are used. Much of the language surrounding old age is borrowed from the world of machines; we talk of 'wear and tear', 'running down', and 'worn out', confirming that ageing people should reduce physical exertion in order to increase their potential lifespan.

This outlook casts doubt on the value of physical exercise, and remains influential with many older people and their carers. As recently as 1970, the opinion of some scientists was that exercise was stressful to the body, with harmful effects similar to those of infections, trauma, and other disease processes (Ashton and Davies,

1986). Such ideas encourage the tendency for old age to become sedentary, dominated by attitudes about physical activity similar to those on retirement, considered by many to be an end of activity, rather than a beginning.

The mechanistic analogy is mistaken. Machines are manufactured with materials not capable of renewal, so degeneration is inevitable. Unlike machines, the body is not created once and for all; the process of cell renewal is part of the biological activity which continually maintains life. Yet the theory is probably more pernicious than this, and misses the essential difference between the constitution of machine, and a living organism (Gore, 1973). Metabolic processes work best in response to the demands made by the body. If the body is not exercised, no demands are made, leading to stagnation. Conversely, exercise encourages the process of renewal, and vitality is thereby enhanced.

Mechanistic ideas linger on. Many older people wonder whether exercise is safe, particularly in relation to the cardiovascular system. These doubts are reinforced by medical practices which intimate that bodily parts do wear out, and that new ones can be transplanted whenever necessary. Such fears are misplaced; physical activity in old age is not only desirable, within personal limitations, but both necessary and beneficial.

Indeed, exercise is considerably healthier than prolonged inactivity. An extreme indication of this can be inferred when enforced inactivity is imposed on the body, for example, when a broken limb is placed in plaster, the muscles waste and weaken, and are returned to normal functioning by exercise. More generally, lack of physical activity is increasingly associated with illness, and particularly with the increase in coronary heart disease. There is mounting evidence, and a growing realization, that exercise is central to good health quite regardless of age, and almost regardless of illness.

Recent interest in physical fitness has not been entirely helpful to older people. Youth-centred ideas are based on the premise that if a little exercise is good, a great deal more must be better, itself linked to the idea that exercise needs to hurt if it is to be beneficial. This is not only incorrect, it can prevent older people from believing that exercise is something in which they can usefully participate. Exercise can, indeed, be taken to extreme limits of physical endurance by young people who wish to develop their strength, power and flexibility; but this level of exercise has a different purpose. For the maintenance of health, rigorous exercise is quite unnecessary, and probably quite wrong for the older individual.

Youthist ideas can represent an enormous mental hurdle for older people, making even the mildest exercise programme appear daunting, and simultaneously worthless. What needs to be recognized is that very little effort is required to maintain an efficient body. Indeed, for the frail, or very unfit, it is sensible to limit exercise. There are three factors to consider: the intensity of exercise, or how hard; the duration of exercise, or how long; and the frequency of exercise, or how often. Most advice suggests that light, but sustained exertion for 10 to 15 minutes a day, three of four times a week, is sufficient, always starting at an easy pace, extending the length and frequency of sessions only as fitness develops.

Individuals who have exercized regularly should not stop because of misguided ageist notions, but continue to the boundaries of their personal limitations, which they are quite capable of sensibly assessing for themselves. Indeed, individuals who are used to regular exercise can suffer more than others if they stop. The benefits of exercise are not long lasting; nor can they be stored from youth and passed to old age. Exercise is a requirement for a lifetime, not to be restricted on the basis of age.

Yet exercise is particularly important for those who have allowed their bodies to become deconditioned. Sagging, overweight bodies, protruding stomachs, with head and shoulders bent forward, all constitute health hazards. Yet if defective posture is a common feature of old age, it is avoidable.

Moreover, the required exercise can be accomplished through the tasks of everyday life, starting with simple activities like sitting and standing, lying and lifting, shaving, washing and feeding, taking a brisk walk rather than using transportation, and using the stairs rather than a lift or escalator. Even reflective recreations, such as painting, are certainly exercises of the mind, but also the body in both the preparation and execution of the task. Dancing is another enjoyable social activity, as well as a gentle form of exercise, that many older people have enjoyed for years, but often abandon on account of age. Moreover, it can be artistic, expressive and creative, and thus therapeutic, whilst not being competitive. It can tone the body, improve posture and circulation, and maintain pelvic mobility. Modern dance therapy aims to help withdrawn people and those who experience difficulty in communication and touch, and so can be particularly useful for older people.

However, it is important for deconditioned people, who plan to embark on exercise, not to rely entirely on exercise to regain fitness. The idea that exercise is the panacea for ill health is both simplistic and naive. The belief that people who spend more time exercising their bodies are healthier, and live longer than others is not necessariliy true. Exercise can promote health, but it does not guarantee it. Exercise should be considered just one part of an overall plan, its value placed in the context of a wider, more holistic view of health. For those who smoke, drink heavily, or eat an unhealthy diet, exercise can be harmful. If the capacity of the lungs is being harmed by inhaled tobacco smoke, it is absurd to seek to improve lung function by exercise. If arteries are being furred up by poor diet, it is nonsense to extend their capacity through exercise. The deterioration in diet, already considered, has occurred simultaneously with the decline of physical exercise, and they should be considered together. Nor does exercise overcome the damage to health caused by the stress and tensions of modern life. All these factors should be addressed when embarking on a programme of exercise relating to personal health.

When these aspects of lifestyle are rectified, exercise can be encouraged as an entirely safe activity. Indeed, when lifestyle factors are improved, the need to exercise can arise quite naturally, even with individuals who have hitherto been sluggish, lethargic and generally lacking in energy.

There is no age beyond which it becomes too late to begin exercising. Nor are there any physical prerequisites. People confined to wheelchairs can exercise to the limits of their capability. Graham (1988) states that all the movements described in her book can be undertaken from a sitting position. Even after illness exercise can be beneficial. Those who have suffered physical impairment, or have lost some degree of physical function, need to exercise either to regain it, or to retain what remains. Doctors used to prescribe long periods of rest after a heart attack, but now patients are encouraged to undertake gentle forms of exercise.

There are clearly some reservations, and some situations where a consultation with a doctor may be advisable. Caution may be required for those who have suffered major joint damage, or who suffer from major heart disease. Any tightness or pain felt in the upper body on taking exercise should be considered a warning sign. Thus, if consulting with the doctor is felt necessary, do so. However, if the medical answer to exercise is 'no', a second opinion should be sought as such a reaction is, in most cases, too uncompromising to be based upon anything but a mechanistic view of bodily requirements.

There are two levels of exercise. Aerobic exercise means literally 'depending on oxygen'. The body uses oxygen to burn fat and carbohydrate stored within the body so that it can release energy to fuel the muscles as quickly as possible. Anaerobic exercise takes over when the level of exercise becomes so intense that the energy released by aerobic metabolism is insufficient to meet the demands of the muscles. The body then releases energy by a rapid breakdown of its stores of body sugar, producing instead lactic acid in the muscles, which eventually produces muscle fatigue and cramp.

For the maintenance of health in old age, it is not necessary to exercise to the point of exhaustion. Aerobic exercise is all that is required, although, at the same time, there is no necessary restriction on this. Whatever activity is chosen, whether this be swimming, cycling, rambling, bowling, fishing, dancing, cricket, golf, yoga or anything else, it needs to be sufficiently brisk to increase heart rate, have an effect on the muscles, and cause moderate breathlessness. This is required quite regardless of the degree of physical fitness. As fitness improves, increased activity will be required to achieve these results, indicating that progress is being made.

THE HEALTH BENEFITS OF EXERCISE

Physical activity is an integral part of being alive, and creates a physiological stimulus to which the whole organism responds positively. There needs to be greater recognition that the maintenance of health depends upon exercise. The hazards of inactivity for older people are substantial, leading to circulatory and joint troubles, lowered resistance to infection, slower recovery from illness or injury, and ultimately to immobility and disability. Indeed, lack of exercise can lead to pathological old age, with all its attendant infirmities. These are the consequences of ageing many people fear, but they are ones that the individual can avoid.

Cardiovascular fitness

A healthy heart is vital to health. The cardiovascular system is literally at the heart of any fitness programme. The heart is a very specialist, robust muscle, and as with any other muscle, exercise is vital to its performance. A strong heart beats as effectively, and as infrequently as possible, in order to circulate sufficient blood to the body. The stroke volume of the heart is calculated by the amount of blood displaced by each contraction. The more blood displaced, the more efficient the heart.

The benefits of exercise arise from the 'training effect' on the heart, reducing heart rate by increasing its efficiency in pumping blood around the body with each contraction. Exercise improves heart and respiratory functioning by reducing blood pressure, purging the arterial system of fatty deposits, regulating blood-sugar levels, controlling body weight, and providing an added means of controlling stress. All these factors reduce susceptibility to heart disease. Exercise is also a useful method of achieving weight loss, and countering obesity, a known health hazard.

Conversely, lack of exercise is one of the main factors contributing to the premature degeneration of the heart, and the circulatory system. There is now irrefutable evidence that exercise offers protection to coronary heart disease (Ashton and Davies, 1986); and it has also been estimated that exercise can halve the death rate of those suffering from hypertension. Exercise protects the heart by increasing the circulation of enzymes that breaks down the fats contained in the blood, leading, in turn, to the manufacture of more fat-carrying particles, called high-density lipoproteins, which carry cholesterol from the tissues to the liver.

Complicated systems exist by which individuals can calculate how much exercise the heart requires, based on the 'target heart rate'. This is the number of beats per minute to which heart rate should be raised. There are several formulas used, but the target figure is calculated by subtracting chronological age from 220 (the theoretical outer limit of heartbeats per minute), then multiplying that figure by 60% if one is unfit, 70% if moderately fit, and 80% if very fit. Yet there is no accepted body of science to support such formulas, which are based on arbitrary assumptions. As Cailliet and Gross (1987) contend, individuals do not need to check their pulse to know that the heart is beating quicker, or to confirm that they are breathless, and this is all that is required by those who wish to exercise for health.

Strength

Loss of strength with ageing is caused more by inactivity than age. The body contains literally billions of muscle cells at birth, and even the longest-surviving individuals are destined to use only a small proportion of them. Ageing does lead to a gradual loss of strength, but not one which needs to be significant. Exercise reduces the loss of muscle fibre, and the capacity of muscles will more than meet the requirements of older people, providing the muscles are kept in good shape. Indeed, if an individual begins to exercise late in life, following years of inactivity, it is quite possible that they can be stronger in old age than in middle age.

Regular activity can slow the physiological deterioration that is often seen as part of normal ageing. Unused muscles degenerate because of insufficient blood reaching them, whilst exercised muscles are able to extract oxygen more efficiently from the blood, and can increase the number of capillaries that supply them, permitting more oxygenated blood to maintain them. Lack of exercise can also dangerously diminish the quality of blood, and its ability to transport essential oxygen and calcium to the muscles. When the supply of these two elements are reduced, muscle fibre loses bulk, and tendons and ligaments become more fragile.

Inactivity causes muscle to be replaced with fat; exercise reverses this, conserves muscle, converting fat tissue into muscle tissue, thereby improving body-tone. Another health benefit then arises from the fact that muscle gain, and fat loss, will lead to a slimmer appearance, improved self-confidence and higher morale.

In order to gain these advantages, the principle of overload is important. This means that the load moved, the number of repetitions done, and the speed of the movement, needs to be progressively increased. Again, it is not necessary to use elaborate techniques or equipment; the weight of the body represents 'load', so at least, initially, general everyday activity is all that is necessary.

Flexibility and mobility

The loss of flexibility and mobility, eventually accompanied with pain, are the greatest deficits experienced by many older people. Mobility is the most important single factor ensuring independence, and its loss is often the direct consequence of inadequate exercise. The problem is not muscle or bone structure, but the cartilage and ligaments which connect the bones at the joints. Cartilage acts as a cushion at the end of every bone entering a joint, whilst ligaments hold the bones in place, guide them in their movement, and restrict them from moving too much. These tissues are vitally important.

Neglected, it shrivels and dies, and makes you stiff and prematurely old in the process. Exercised regularly and properly, it springs back to life, restoring that youthful suppleness you imagined had gone for ever.

(Cailliet and Gross, 1987)

Cartilage needs to be regularly compressed, although not too harshly. The ligaments need to be regularly stretched; but not overstretched. If this is not done, the tissues will gradually lose their flexibility, and the joints will stiffen. Such stiffness is only partly due to ageing; it is mainly the consequence of inactivity, associated with a sedentary lifestyle, and the ageist expectations of older people. Exercise maintains joint flexibility, suppleness, strength and nimbleness, and has been shown to have a positive effect on degenerative arthritis. An associated benefit is that more flexible, active muscles enhances reaction time.

Another direct effect of exercise on the ageing process is to conserve the strength and density of the bones, and to combat, or even reverse, the onset of the crippling disease, osteoporosis, in which bone become progressively thinner and more fragile. Exercise helps by restoring the natural balance of the bone, probably by placing it under mechanical stress, and triggering the process of bone renewal.

Exercise and the mind

Fitness has mental as well as physical benefits. The mind, like muscle, deteriorates if not used. Engaging our minds, confidently and enthusiastically, is closely connected with how we feel physically. The positive benefits for a healthy mind arising from physical exercise arise from the personal experience of many people, and studies reveal that exercise produces clearer thinking, helps people to feel more optimistic, and can reduce susceptibility to depression in old age. Whilst other processes are also involved, most psychiatrists would acknowledge that physical fitness is an important component of good mental health, enabling the use of mental faculties more acutely and energetically.

These psychological benefits can arise from several factors: organized exercise can bring people together in groups. It can give people more control over their own bodies; and it can increase stamina, allowing people to engage in more activity. There are also known physiological changes which arise from exercise. Exercise modifies brain chemistry by producing a group of hormones collectively called endorphins, a pain killer similar in their effects to morphine, but produced naturally by the body. These can relieve pain, not just by acting on the pain mechanism, but by inhibiting the emotional response to pain. It has been suggested that mental attitudes can themselves affect the secretion of endorphins and thereby the perception of disease.

In these ways, exercise has many beneficial effects on the physical condition of older people, and the illnesses and conditions that affect them, including impaired circulation, respiration, hormonal balance, joint mobility, nervous and muscular co-ordination, blood chemistry and digestion. It can assist in the natural production of insulin within the body to deal with diabetes. In healthy people, regular physical activity helps to keep bodily systems unimpaired, and to continue functioning properly (Gore, 1973).

Many conditions which are considered typical features of decline in old age are, in fact, the features of an inactive old age, not the result of ageing itself. Research suggests that regular, moderate exercise can not only retard the many physiological declines associated with ageing, but can sometimes reverse them. With so many advantages for the maintenance of health, Cailliet and Gross (1987) asked whether any allopathic drug could provide so many advantages, do so naturally, and completely without side-effects; it is a legitimate question.

The problem is that the more unfit individuals become, the harder it is for them to start exercising. As exercise appears to be less possible, so it becomes less likely that exercise will recommend itself, or be recommended to them. The result is that exercise is rarely considered as a potential method of maintaining health in old age.

POSTURE: THE ALEXANDER TECHNIQUE

Good posture is an important element in the maintenance of health. Looking good makes us feel good. Feeling good makes us take care of our appearance, which is not simply a physical matter, but an expression of how we feel. The stooping gait, so often associated with older people, not only makes people look old, but makes them feel old, and encourages them to function like 'old people'.

Western medicine has overlooked the importance of correct posture, especially in the head and neck (Stanway, 1982). Retaining, or regaining, good posture should be a primary objective in modifying the effects of ageing. There are correct and incorrect ways to stand, sit, bend, lift and walk. When bad habits arise, the strain of these everyday movements can be damaging. The origin of poor posture can often be traced to childhood, exacerbated by sedentary occupations and lifestyle, with the major problems becoming apparent only in old age. Cailliet and Gross (1987) suggest that poor posture begins when the head begins to droop forward, imperceptibly at first, more noticeably later. As the head weighs between 10 and 15 lb, this change alters the entire balance of the body. Other muscles and ligaments have to lengthen or shorten in order to compensate, leading to losses in the range of movement, as joints can no longer function as intended. Posture becomes curved: the shoulders hunch, the head slumps further, the back stoops, the chest sags, the stomach protrudes, and we lose height.

There are also known connections between emotional stress and posture. Emotionally, tension is transformed into physical tension, for the reaction to tension is to flex or contract the muscles. Muscles which are constantly contracted ultimately produce an adaptive shortening of connective tissue, with muscles, ligaments and tendons becoming less elastic. This can eventually lead to restricted mobility, an inefficient body, and ultimately to painful joint dysfunction.

Bad posture can cause muscular aches and pains, and increased pain and discomfort in the joints, particularly in the back and lower spine. The prevalence of stiffness and pain in old age emphasizes the importance of correct posture. There is nothing more crippling and debilitating than backache, making it difficult to walk, or even to sit or lie down.

Such mis-use of the body can lead to dis-ease. Contracted muscles demand additional nourishment, but the physical tension can restrict blood supply to them. Slumping posture can also cause the constriction of the chest and shoulder muscles, reducing breathing function and oxygen intake. Bad posture distorts the stomach, lungs and other organs, making it harder for them to function efficiently, and even increasing the risk of chest infections and indigestion.

The effects of the Alexander technique in remedying postural problems can be particularly helpful. The technique is not a medical treatment, but a form of personal re-education which seeks to point out bad habits, and replace them with more natural movements. It aims to treat, and prevent, a range of disorders, essentially through a system of postural change, based on the premise that people, throughout their lives, develop habits which are unnatural, unhealthy and, ultimately, lead to pain and disease. The technique seeks to help the individual rediscover and recondition basic posture and movement patterns.

126

Common movements, such as walking, sitting and talking, are usually taken for granted. There is a tendency to become lazy and develop bad habits. Such movements are, however, very complex actions involving many thousands of nerves and muscles. Over a number of years, the body rebalances itself, often incorrectly, subjecting it to strains for which it is unfitted. By the time most people reach adult life, many harmful postural habits have developed, leading to mental and physical tension, altering the expansion capability of the chest, impairing breathing, and creating pain in all parts of the body, especially in old age.

Everyone can benefit, although Hope (1989) suggests that the technique is best suited to the thinker or intellectual rather than the individual simply looking for a period of relaxation and enjoyment. Older people, who have had more time to develop and habitualize postural defects, can find it particularly helpful. The Alexander technique suggests that many people have to alter postural habits, and replace them with new, more constructive physical and mental attitudes. It therefore requires more personal commitment to change than other manipulative therapies; but with older people, in continuous pain, this need not present an insuperable problem.

Several lessons from a competent Alexander technician can quickly change postural habits. Thereafter, the individual can continue at home, preventing many kinds of pain by a method entirely without side-effects. People have found that their movements quickly become smoother, easier, lighter and faster, and it has also been found to increase the general sense of well-being. It is specifically valuable for postural problems, breathing troubles, asthma, speech defects, bone or muscle disorders, and severe low-back and sciatic pain; but is also useful for those suffering from high blood pressure, spastic colon, trigeminal neuraliga, osteoarthritis and asthma.

RELAXATION, REST AND SLEEP

Tension can be as damaging to health as any bacteria or virus, ultimately causing major harm to health. Unrelieved tension and anxiety can initially produce reactions ranging from headaches, skin disorders, and failing eyesight but, subsequently, it can become a prime factor in hypertension, heart disease, and many other serious illnesses.

Learning to relax is the best antidote to the health damage caused by physical and mental tension. The best tranquillizer is the ability to relax, sleep and rest, not those obtained by medical prescription.

Moreover, there are many techniques designed to assist relaxation, seeking to teach the individual how to avoid muscle contraction. By learning instead to consciously develop muscular relaxation, the individual can release the nervous tension that contributes to the ageing process and, in doing so, can also lower blood pressure, and slow heart and breathing rates.

To avoid the complaint of inconsistency, the need for relaxation and rest needs to be differentiated from the need for exercise. If inactivity is to be avoided, why do we need rest and sleep at all? The distinction surrounds the significant biological difference between inactivity, and rest after effort. Exercise assists relaxation by producing endorphins, the natural tranquillizing hormones which act as both painkiller and relaxant. Exercise is also known to produce an electrical effect on the neurological connections in the muscles, which also relaxes them. In this way, older people can be assisted in relaxing through the mechanical, chemical and electrical reactions arising from exercise.

Many older people seek the rest and sleep that arises from a lack of physical activity, the need for sleep arising from a tired, depressed or bored brain. Many people feel tired at the end of an uneventful, inactive day, retire early to bed, wake early, potter around, feel tired, have a sleep after lunch, and again feel tired by evening. This represents an attempt to sleep through habit or boredom rather than fulfilling a requirement of the body; sleep becomes a way of passing time. A lack of fitness increases the need for sleep because of the inefficient operation, and poor recovery rate of the body.

This makes inactivity the basis for much insomnia in old age. Normally, it is the expenditure of energy through activity that produces the need to rest. Relaxation and sleep then fulfil the body's need for recovery, and to supply extra energy for future use. It is the rest which follows exercise that the body requires; sleep after inactivity is not equivalent to sleep after exertion (Gore, 1973).

Insomnia can be a serious matter for older people, ultimately affecting physical and mental efficiency. Individuals need to identify the factors that keep them awake, what makes their sleep fitful, or wakes them too soon. Healthy people tend to need less sleep. The body may need rest when it is tired, but has no use for sleep otherwise. The need for sleep therefore varies with personal circumstances.

Depression is a major cause of insomnia, often leaving the individual lying awake, tense with worry, the mind unable to cope. Even when sleep is possible, the individual often awakes feeling gloomy and downhearted. The ability to awake at a reasonable hour, feeling good, and ready for the day ahead is something that many older people are quite unable to do.

Other causes of insomnia are more straightforward, such as drinking coffee, strong tea, cocoa or other stimulants, particularly late at night. If so, it is simply remedied by abstinence, or by substituting herbal teas, such as camomile, which aid sleep. The standard medical reaction to sleeplessness, hypnotic drugs, are a poor substitute for proper exercise. They are effective only for short periods, after which increased doses to compensate can lead to habituation, whilst usually failing to improve sleep patterns. Many older people use alcohol to achieve the same purpose, a more expensive, less effective and, ultimately, a more addictive response.

YOGA AND OLDER PEOPLE

There are many non-medical or alternative medical responses to the physical aspects of health in older age. Indeed, there are a confusing number of fitness programmes, most of them paying scant regard to the special needs of older people. Whilst some might acknowledge that older people should not exercise as rigorously as younger people, most suggest the same basic approach to exercise for all age groups. Yet without question, the most valuable, comprehensive approach to the physical aspects of health is yoga.

Yoga is a physical, mental and spiritual discipline which dates back some 6000 years. Yoga means union, and is based on concept of the union of body, mind and spirit, which yogic tradition says cannot be separated. It developed from ancient intuitions concerning the postures, methods of breathing, and activity that were beneficial to physical and mental health. Modern research is beginning to verify these discoveries, and many older people by practising yogic methods of moving, stretching and breathing, have found that it is possible to eradicate aches and pains, and increase suppleness and energy. Many claim that it can even delay the signs of ageing.

It is possible for everyone to practise yoga. It is not necessary to be able to twist in all directions, stand on your head, or sit on the floor with your legs tied in knots. All that is required of the individual is the ability to move to whatever extent possible. Yoga involves stretching, not straining; gentle releasing, not forcing to reach a given position; and relaxing the body to enable greater flexibility. It can be practised at home, although attendance at a class is always recommended.

Nor is yoga necessarily a mystical art. The 'higher' purposes contained within yogic philosophy discourage many people who believe that it is a form of religion that imposes its own system of beliefs and values. This does not need to be so. How many of these underlying Hindu beliefs are taken up depends entirely on the individual, and can be completely disregarded.

There are a number of yoga pathways, each seeking to bring unity between the spiritual and bodily self. Yoga is not strictly a system of exercise. Posture, breathing and meditation are its three main ingredients, alongside the bodily positions, called *asanas*, from which the body derives the discipline which enables it to observe the required rigidity with the minimum of physical effort. When correctly executed, the *asanas* free the body from minor discomforts, thus allowing the mind the tranquillity essential for deep meditation. It seeks to get all aspects of the body and mind working in harmony, thereby overcoming the unsatisfactory dualism of dominant Western philosophy.

The advantage of yoga for older people is that it will not cause exhaustion or strain, like many other forms of physical exercise, and is particularly adaptable to individual circumstances as it relies on slow, smooth movements. Brown (1988) has developed a gentle, complete and balanced system of yoga in which the basic postures have been adapted, and more time allowed to accomplish them. She testifies that many of her older students have become excellent adverts for the benefits of yoga. Kent (1985) explains how yoga can be used by disabled people as a self-help method.

As an aid to good health, yoga is to be recommended. The therapeutic effects of meditative practices generally are encouraged by many alternative therapists, and even by some medical practitioners. Yet medicine has hardly begun to examine the benefits claimed by yoga. There is said to be an effect on the hormonal systems important for health in old age. Some yoga postures, for example, the twists and stomach contractions, are thought to stimulate hormonal activity, and to maintain and extend their functioning. This includes the sexual glands, yoga being said to increase sexual vitality and energy. The inverse postures, for example, the head stand or shoulder stand, are said to be important for longevity, arising from increased blood circulation to the brain, which stimulates two small glands, the hypothalamus and pituitary, which control the activity of most of the other hormone-producing glands in the body.

Yoga breathing exercises seek to help the individual develop the conscious use of the lungs and rib cage, changing it from a haphazard and often inefficient event, to one which is actually directed to a purpose. This can be used for developing the unused capacity of the lungs, or for people who suffer form bronchitis, asthma and other chest complaints. Yoga can be particularly helpful with asthma attacks, assisting through a programme of postures, relaxation, internal cleansing and breathing.

Yoga also seeks to develop good posture, and so can be helpful to the aches, strains and pains common to many older people. Good posture not only makes you feel better in yourself, but also puts less strain on muscles and joints, and on cramped internal organs, particularly the lungs. Yoga is helpful with arthritis sufferers by working on the muscles which surround an affected joint, keeping them in good condition, and helping to protect and support the joint, and improve circulation. Brown (1988) claimed that her most encouraging results came from arthritis sufferers.

Yoga also recognizes the importance of responding to the stresses of life, and thus leads to health through relaxation. Yoga relaxation has a very specific purpose: to create stillness in body and mind so that the individual is clear to concentrate, leading to the highly valued state of meditaton. Yoga pays particular attention to concentration, the focusing of attention on an object whilst at the same time being aware of other distractions, and to meditation, when awareness is focused solely on the object of concentration. The benefit of this is that the 'absent mindedness' so often associated with old age is not due to ageing, or the death of brain cells, but is the consequence of inadequate exercise of the brain.

Yoga can contribute to the physical, mental and spiritual well-being of older people, with evidence that yoga can help osteoporosis, perhaps because regular appropriate exercise on yogic lines has even been found to help build up bones that have become weaker, or demineralized. Yoga relaxation can help manage hypertension, by actively lowering blood-pressure.

9

Alternative medicine: the fall and rise of traditional medical practice

Providing reasonable care is taken, the body will keep itself healthy, and when it does fall ill, will usually heal itself. The need for medical assistance, even in old age, will be limited to those times when imbalances within the body develop to an extent that the natural immune system cannot cope. When this happens, the healing process can be helped by many forms of medical assistance.

In deciding who to consult at these times, the social and political confirmation of allopathy, alongside its ready availability, usually ensures that it is to the conventional doctor that we normally call upon first. However, a wider knowledge of the available sources of medical help might lead to quite a different decision.

Alternative medicine, in its many forms, has been castigated as primitive and unscientific by the conventional medical establishment, neither doing justice to these therapies, nor to veracity. This is not new. Parliament was often petitioned by physicians who bewailed the 'worthless and presumptuous women who usurp the profession', demanding fines and imprisonment for women practising medicine (Mitchell, 1984). The medieval persecution of witches was often based on accusations that women could cure illness. The Church denounced non-professional healing as equivalent to heresy: 'If a woman dare cure without having studied, she is a witch and must die'. Usually, these women were not accused of ineffective or dangerous treatment; their crime was to offer remedies for those seeking contraception, abortion, or to ease the pain of labour; they did not have to do harm – to heal was sufficient.

Alternative practitioners are no longer burnt at the stake, but centuries of medical knowledge and expertise continues to be systematically disparaged as 'unscientific', or based upon ignorance and superstition. Fulder (1983) has produced a more recent view of the social opposition facing non-allopathic medical practice, presenting a picture of medical resistance, legal restraints, and bureaucratic obstacles. Yet once most people depended entirely upon these old, disparaged medicines, and they were more favoured than the 'new' scientific medicine, which was feared and hated by most people. What were the reasons for this change?

The social disruption of the Agrarian and Industrial Revolutions played an important role. Herbalism, the oldest and most widespread form of medical treatment, was based in rural villages, and not readily available in cities. The knowledge of local herbs and plants did not easily transfer to the new, industrialized areas, and the disrupted populations were soon removed from their close connections with the land.

Allopathic medicine, based on science and chemicals, was more at home in urban areas, and seemed to be both more exciting, exotic, and heroic in its effects. Many drugs were developed from exotic plants from India, China and America, linked with stories of wondrous properties. Others came from highly toxic substances, usually mercury based, such as calomel, scammony, antimony, sublimate and laudanum, whose action on the body was extreme. Indeed, toxic activity became everything. If a drug could be seen working on the body, it must be effective. Allopathy represents a 'heroic' approach to medicine, identified in the past by bleeding, mustard plasters, purges and highly toxic drugs, which often produced instant, dramatic results, but often with lethal consequences. In comparison, herbal remedies were usually gentle and slow acting. The herbs that survived longest were those which were known to be active purges, such as rhubarb, senna, castor oil, and jalap (Griggs, 1981).

Traditional medicine became old-fashioned and commonplace. Herbalism remained available in rural communities, prescribed by unqualified, older women, and became associated with poor people. The medicine of qualified doctors was available to those who could afford their services. In time, traditional methods were ridiculed by the wealthy, and the poor wanted access to the rich man's medicine. After all, it had to be better; why else would they pay for it (Mitchell, 1984)?

The rising popularity of allopathy was also based on its inclination to absolve the individual from personal responsibility, establishing health as something within the gift of doctors. To live wildly and be returned to health is a popular notion, one that allopathy has effectively promoted.

The assumption of scientific progress also contributed to the decline of traditional medicine. Although based upon centuries of empirical practice and observation, people were led to believe that allopathic medicine was more knowledgeable, and more sophisticated. Nor was this just a medical conspiracy; Griggs (1981) commented on the curious and depressing truth that the aspiration of physicians to dispense powerful and active drugs has only been equalled by the desire of patients to have powerful drugs administered to them.

Resentment towards the medical establishment, whose fees had placed professional care out of the reach of poorer people, evaporated with the introduction of national health insurance, and ultimately the National Health Service. The 1911 National Insurance Act refused to incorporate other forms of medicine. Although it did not prohibit benefit for those attending herbalists, it became virtually impossible for insured people to do so. Social legislation made everyone financially dependent upon allopathic medicine.

A similar process took place in the USA, when the Flexnor Report 'united' the various schools of medicine. Ostensibly established in the interests of unity, it proved to be the *coup de grâce* for 'irregular medical schools'. Henceforth, no medical school could exist without American Medical Association approval, which soon promoted drug-oriented, allopathic medicine, effectively eliminating all other forms.

Despite the growing public consciousness of the limitations of conventional medicine, alternative medicine remains a fringe activity. Until their recent re-emergence, some alternative medical therapies were almost entirely lost, and without doubt a considerable body of former knowledge and experience has irretrievably gone. The medical establishment continues to dismiss alternative approaches, and does so with a persistence and energy which suggests that dominant attitudes have less to do with superiority, and more with a self-interested oppression of rivals. Yet as evidence mounts of the relative inefficiency of allopathy, and it is perceived that general health is not improving, recognition of medical limitations will spread, and the need for different approaches will increase.

The revival and reappraisal of alternative medicine is the result. Its benefits for older people have never been closely examined, but emanates from the underlying philosophy that the body can, and usually does, heal itself. Alternative medicine seeks to 'heal' rather than to 'cure', the bolder term favoured by allopathy. Many therapies are designed for self-help, so that once their procedures have been mastered, older people can practise them independently, within the security of their home, leading to more personal control over their health. Fulder (1988) suggests that there are five principal tenets shared by alternative medicines, each strikingly different from the tenets of conventional medicine.

First, that therapy starts with a full constitutional and biographical picture of the individual, with treatment seeking to realign and restore imbalances, defects, and destructive patterns by determining why they have arisen within the individual.

Second, that the artificial barriers between the mind, body and spirit, are absent. Lifestyle, attitude, caste of mind, vital energy and posture are all considered relevant in treatment.

Third, that they all use the broader definition of health, which includes complete physical and mental well-being, encompassing poor vitality and low resistance.

Fourth, that they are best suited to treat the chronic, psychogenic and organic diseases for which individual resistance and health is a key to recovery.

Fifth, that all therapies have the goal of self-healing, are generally harmless, and utilize non-toxic remedies.

There are many forms of alternative medicine, most of them relatively simple, effective, harmless and holistic. It is the benefits that older people can gain from them that now require consideration. It is not possible to personally recommend them all, so in the subsequent sections I am indebted to the authors listed in the References, and to the various national organizations who have provided information, and whose addresses are given in the Appendix.

NATUROPATHY: *MEDICUS CURAT, NATURA SANAT* (THE DOCTOR TREATS, BUT NATURE HEALS)

Natural healing has the most distinct alternative medical philosophy, and the one most critically opposed to allopathic medicine. It is probably the least intrusive strategy medically, but certainly the most interventionist socially. It believes that individuals are responsible for their own health, discounts easy medical solutions, and imposes tough choices between health and personal lifestyle.

Naturopathy is based on three main principles (Benjamin, 1936). The most fundamental is that all disease arises from toxins and waste materials that accumulate within the body. Naturopaths argue that disease can be cured only by enabling the body to discharge these toxic wastes. Many aspects of modern life can cause disharmony, but the main cause of toxic accumulation is malnutrition. Whilst diet formerly consisted of grains, nuts, raw fruit, fresh vegetables, proteins and pure water, it now consists of refined, devitalized grains, highly salted nuts, frozen or canned fruits and vegetables, and complex proteins, many poisoned by chemicals. These are augmented by harmful beverages, such as coffee, tea and alcohol.

Whilst earlier naturopaths believed that toxic material arose mainly from lifestyle factors, particularly diet, it is now acknowledged that toxicity also has psychological and environmental roots, including factors such as stress, pollution, poverty and the lack of physical exercise. It recognizes that the air we breath is no longer pure, and that drugs, cigarettes and exposure to many toxic chemicals serve to increase human vulnerability. Emotions, such as fear, anxiety, hate, self-pity and resentment, are also recognized as factors which can upset digestion, blood flow and hormonal balance.

The second principle is that the body works constantly in the direction of positive health, that the 'vital force' within each individual steadily works towards self-cleansing and self-repair. The body's immune system mobilizes antibodies to suppress disease, and eliminates unwanted toxic substances via the bowels, kidneys, skin and lungs. Diarrhoea and vomiting deal with the digestive system; sneezing and coughing rid the respiratory system of irritants; sweating removes toxins through the skin; mucous secretions are extruded through the nose and mouth; and menstruation performs an additional eliminative function for women. Inflammation and swelling localize infections until the body's blood and lymph supply removes the waste material. High temperature creates a less favourable environment for foreign bacteria and viruses to increase.

Natural therapy considers all these processes to be corrective and eliminative, positive action to remove impediments to good health. The aim of natural healing is to support these internal forces rather than regarding the body as helpless in the face of disease, and in need of medical assistance.

Yet when natural eliminative channels are overburdened, and can no longer cope with the constant subjection to toxins and waste materials, illness is the result, with acute disease striking at the weakest, most vulnerable part of the body. Yet even here the interpretation of illness is different. Such illness is considered to be the activity of the body attempting to re-establish balance. The symptoms of acute illness are regarded as the self-repairing efforts of the body to restore health, an intelligent response to rid itself of unwanted waste materials, and repair injured tissue. The fever is not an illness, but a method utilized by the body to increase metabolic rate, and the circulation of blood and lymph, which all speed the removal of toxins by the body's more complicated defence, such as white blood cells and antibodies.

This places natural therapy in direct conflict with allopathic medicine, which seeks not only to suppress the activity the body, but imposes additional burdens by introducing drugs to an already over-toxified body.

This is important when considering the third principle of naturopathy, which states that the body can return itself to a state of health, provided that the correct assistance is given. This is based on the premise that health is best maintained by energizing the body's ability to protect, regulate, adjust and heal itself.

Naturopathy considers *chronic* illness to be the result of medical efforts to suppress the physiological efforts of the body to cleanse itself. If the symptoms of actue illness are repressed, then chronic disease will eventually result. The 'cure' of acute disease through allopathic drugs or surgery forces the toxins, which the body is seeking to eliminate, deeper into the system. It is this build-up of toxicity in the vital organs and structures of the body which forms the basis of future chronic disease, ultimately striking when bodily resistance is low. The form chronic disease takes will depend upon the individual's bodily constitution, and hereditary tendencies, but the basic principle is that all chronic disease, regardless of its form, originates from the suppression of acute illness.

Allopathic medicine suppresses important warning signs that require investigation. Pain, for example, is a natural mechanism, which draws attention to a problem that the body can no longer tolerate, a warning that further neglect may cause more serious injury. Pain-killers rid the body of pain, thus allowing more serious, longer-term dangers to be ignored.

Naturopathy considers that the body sometimes requires assistance to recover from illness. Diet is usually the primary element in naturopathic treatment, both by adjusting eating habits and/or periods of fasting. Fasting is one of the oldest natural therapies known. Animals always stop eating when unwell, laying quietly, preferably alone, drinking sufficient fluid to prevent dehydration. Fasting enables the body to compensate for illness. Energy is redirected from normal day-to-day processes, such as the digestion and assimilation of food, to the elimination of toxins through natural channels. Although fasting can produce some rather unpleasant side-effects, including halitosis, diarrhoea, vomiting and headache, these are recognized as the body's efforts to detoxify itself, indicators that the treatment is working. They soon disappear, alongside the initial hunger.

The value of naturopathic philosophy to older people arises from the remarkable powers of tolerance and adaptation of the body. Younger people can cope with many social, environmental and self-imposed threats which place the body under pressure, for it is still sufficiently resilient to withstand serious illness or disease. With ageing, increasing penalties are exacted. Youthful tolerance declines with regular abuse. The acute illnesses of childhood and middle age will have been suppressed, only to reappear in chronic forms in later years. The older body will be increasingly unable to cope with the toxicity to which it is subjected. The degenerative diseases which characterize the lives of older people, and which are so often discounted as the inevitable result of ageing, are the long-term result of misguided social, personal and medical practice.

The medical philosophy of naturopathy is not widely accepted or, indeed, known. However, if after years of allopathic treatment, the older individual continues to suffer the pain and disability of chronic disease, it is a philosophy that is surely worth testing out. It is an excellent self-help therapy, except perhaps for the longer fasts, which require careful monitoring. It is also an inexpensive, sometimes a cost-free therapy. The availability of naturopaths is limited, but they can be found by writing to national organizations who will provide the addresses of local practitioners.

HOMEOPATHY: *SIMILIS SIMILIBUS CURENTUR* (LET LIKE BE CURED BY LIKE)

Homeopathy is a complete system of medicine, based on the principle that agents which would produce certain signs and symptoms when ingested normally, also assist in curing disease which produces similar signs and symptoms. This is entirely opposite to the principles of allopathic medicine, which applies drugs which produce a contrary reaction in the body. For instance, fevers are treated allopathically with drugs which lower the body temperature, but homeopathically with remedies which raise body temperature. Diarrhoea is treated allopathically with drugs that produce constipation, but homeopathically by remedies which produce diarrhoea.

Unlike many forms of alternative medicine, homeopathy is a relatively recent development. Dr Samuel Hahnemann, a German physician, first developed the practice in the early nineteenth century, since when it has become increasingly popular, without becoming anything other than a 'fringe' activity. Despite the success of homeopathy it continues to be scorned by the medical establishment. As recently as 1986, a British Medical Association report rejected homeopathy, considering its 'minimum dose' ideas as irrational.

Homeopathy, like naturopathy, is based on the principle that the body can cope with most illness without assistance, and that the symptoms of disease indicate that the body is attempting to heal itself. Rather than fighting or suppressing these symptoms, homeopathy seeks to support and encourage them, thereby stimulating the disease-resistant qualities of the body. Homeopathic preparations, called remedies, are extracts of naturally occurring substances, mainly herbs and plants, but also animal material, and natural chemicals. Many of the substances used are poisonous in their natural state, but unlike allopathic drugs, remedies never produce toxic side-effects.

The reason for this is the principle of minimum dose, which whilst simple to describe, its efficacy is difficult to explain. The basic substance of each remedy is pulped and triturated, and called the mother tincture. This is progressively diluted by a process called succussion to produce a particular potency. This process of dilution, or potentization, produces the mystery, for as the remedy is successively triturated and succussed, few if any molecules of the original mother tincture remain. Yet the higher the potency, the fewer molecules of the original substance remaining in the remedy, the more the impact the remedy has on illness. There has never been an entirely adequate explanation for this, hence one of the difficulties homeopathy has is gaining credibility. I once prescribed a homeopathic remedy for my step-daughter, and her father had the tablet analysed, perhaps in the belief that I intended to poison her. He was apparently told that the tablet was entirely inert, completely harmless, nothing more than a placebo. Perhaps the explanation is that remedies work in alliance with the body's own homeostatic system, rather than trying to over-ride them. After all, inoculation works on the same principle.

Homeopathy provides remedies for all forms of illness. It is also a comparatively simple and stable form of medicine. There are probably over 2000 separate remedies available, each in many different potencies: but about 20 remedies are capable of coping with most everyday problems.

The prescription of remedies is not disease specific, but person specific. Homeopathy treats the individual, not the illness. Two people suffering from the same illness might receive entirely different remedies, in different potencies, from the same homeopath. Not only are the diagnostic symptoms considered, but also the personality, temperament and disposition of the individual concerned. Likes, dislikes, the effects of heat and cold, and many other factors are all considered before a remedy is prescribed.

Homeopathic prescription is not considered without regard to individual lifestyle. The homeopath would not prescribe a remedy, even if it was thought to be the correct one, if it was known that the condition resulted from lifestyle factors, such as stress, bad diet or lack of exercise. Correction of these factors would be the primary focus of treatment, with the remedy being used primarily to aid recovery. The future maintenance of health would depend upon personal decisions and choices regarding the use and abuse of the body.

Again, the individual focus of homeopathy has made its effectiveness very difficult to verify. Most science is based on objectivity. The subjectivity of homeopathy, through its primary focus on the individual, does not conform to the principles of science. Many would say, however, that it conforms more closely to the needs of individual people. The value of medical intervention should not depend upon scientific verification, however useful this may be, but with the results it produces for sick people. There are an increasing number of people who can verify its effectiveness. Moreover, because of potentization, homeopathy is an entirely safe form of medicine, without side effects; the reason for its non-acceptability within scientific circles is the very reason for its attraction to people who no longer wish to be associated with iatrogenic disease.

The potential value of homeopathy to older people arises from their vulnerability to the iatrogenic consequences of allopathic medicine, largely arising from decreased kidney and liver function, which reduces their body's ability to cope with drug toxicity. Any form of medicine which offers to treat illness without harmful side-effects must be a considerable advantage for older people.

The non-toxicity of the remedies also enables safe self-medication by older people, removed from the dangers commonly associated with allopathic drugs. Homeopaths do not generally disagree with this, certainly for minor complaints, but it is important that the individual has some knowledge of homeopathy, for, otherwise, remedies can be taken without effect, and eventually dismissed as useless. Treating more serious illness is best done through consultation with a homeopath, to gain the benefit from greater knowledge, and more detailed prescribing ability gained from professional training and practice.

HERBAL MEDICINE: *VIS MEDICATRIX NATURAE* – THE HEALING POWER OF NATURE

Herbal medicine is the oldest form of therapy. *Vis medicatrix naturae* is certainly an Hippocratic idea; the Chinese used herbs in an extensive and sophisticated way 5000 years ago; and evidence from an Iranian grave excavation dated to 60 000 years ago, indicates that it was practised then. Most villages in Britain and Europe in the Middle Ages had a 'wise woman' whose knowledge of the healing properties of local herbs had been passed down over centuries.

Wild animals instinctively seek out plants which will supply the nutrients they need, and unerringly avoid those which will poison them. Humanity has lost this instinctual knowledge of the value of plants, and during the last two hundred years, has also systematically discounted its own verbal and written heritage in favour of the new science. This loss has only recently been halted and reversed, despite the continued opposition of the allopathic medical establishment.

Herbalism is another complete form of medicine, although it is probably more complex and varied in practice, and less uniformly understood than any other type of medicine. Herbalism involves the preparation of all manner of plants, including roots, leaves, stems and seeds. Preparations can take the form of medicines, ointments and teas. There are many thousands of plants used in herbal medicine, and many thousands more which have probably never been investigated. The complexity of the medicinal value of plants is amazing. Even the same plant growing in a different soil has distinct constituent qualities. It is even claimed that the same plant, picked at different times of the year, or even at different times of the day, also varies in medicinal qualities.

It is this complexity, and the lack of standardization, which medical science finds hard to accept. There is an immense amount of information available about the health value of plants, but little consistent agreement over what remedies to use for particular disorders. Nor has there been any consistent attempt to develop a basic philosophy, or any universally accepted fundamental concepts (Fulder, 1988). This can be extremely confusing to anyone who wishes to use herbal medicine, particularly those who believe that there should be a one-to-one relationship between a specific illness, and a remedy.

Herbs can also be used singly, or in combinations, each being prepared for the general improvement of health of a particular individual, not just the relief of symptoms. Fulder (1988) identified three essential therapeutic features of the herbal remedy.

First, they have challenging qualities which tend to provoke a number of protective responses from the body.

Second, they adjust the body process, exhibiting a normalizing, supportive action on organs and tissues, acting almost like foods rather than medicines.

Third, herbal remedies are eliminatory, being particularly good at improving the action of the bowels, kidneys, lungs and sweat glands.

The potential value of herbalism to older people arises from its ability to cure all forms of illness. Herbal remedies can be categorized according to their effects on the body, just as allopathic drugs are, with anti-inflammatories, antispasmodics, anticatarrhals, diuretics, expectorants and laxatives, although their gentler action supports and encourages the work of the body rather than takes over from it. Although it is probably best used as a preventative technique to maintain health, to treat minor ailments, or the early stages of more serious disease, this can probably be said about all medical techniques. Some of the ailments that can be treated herbally have been outlined by Stanway (1982).

- Bronchitis – comfrey.
- Constipation – alder, blackthorn, fennel, liquorice, molasses, prunes, slippery elm.
- Fatigue – agrimony, marjoram, peppermint, rose hips.
- Gout – colchicum, hyssop, juniper.
- Headache – camomile, lavender, mint, poppy.
- Insomnia– aniseed, bergamot, hops, valerian.
- Rheumatism – tonic tea of agrimony, camomile, ground elder, hyssop, mugwort, onion, rosemary.

Herbalism is not a simple matter. The vast number of plants, their medicinal qualities, how to recognize and prepare them, and in what way, and in what quantity, are all matters which require considerable knowledge. As a form of self-medication, herbalism can be restricted by this, but it also has many advantages. Plants grow everywhere, and it is the plentiful supply of local plants that makes herbalism immediately available. Drugs from local plants are believed to bestow the most medical value to the individual; they are difficult for drug companies to patent, and are thus inexpensive. Despite the complexities, herbalism is probably used more often as a form of self-medication by individuals who have taken time to study local plants and their medicinal qualities. This is the herbal tradition, and for older people who have the interest and time, it can be not only an engrossing study, but a very healthy use of spare time.

The beginner can start by selecting a few, readily available herbs, such as burdock, dandelion, horseradish, parsley, garlic, camomile, comfrey, meadowsweet, or a number of any other locally available plants, and learn about their properties (Inglis and West, 1983). Hoffman (1990) gives a similar list of commonly used herbs. Anyone wishing to make use of herbs for curative purposes should be aware that there can be minor side-effects, such as irritations; but they do not have the toxic effects of allopathic drugs.

For the less adventurous, herbal preparations can be obtained from local health-food shops, and it is usually possible to find a good local herbalist for advice. It should also be remembered that herbs can be a form of health-giving enjoyment when taken in the form of teas. Herbal teas not only produce beneficial results for health, but also substitute for conventional Indian teas and coffee, which are both high in caffeine, and consumed in great quantities by many older people to the detriment of their health.

AROMATHERAPY

Aromatherapy is part of an ancient natural healing tradition which utilizes the health-giving effects of the essential oils of plants, and their aroma. These are imparted to the body through massage, baths and teas, to revive, restore and heal. It seeks to combine sensual pleasure with medicine. Whether the objective is to relax tired muscles, reduce stress, enhance sensuality, cure minor ailments, such as headaches, aches and pains, or just to enjoy the pleasure of scented massage, aromatherapy is safe, effective and enjoyable.

The essential oils are extracted from the bark, roots, stalks, leaves, flowers and resins of plants. They are utilized through massage, baths, inhalation, teas and other techniques which seek to revive, restore and heal the body. The application of the oils is undertaken princi-pally by massage, during which the aromatic essences are inhaled, and the healing qualities of the oil penetrate through the skin. These are the three healing routes of aromatherapy, although the processes through which aromatic essences work remain uncertain.

In aromatherapy massage, essential oils, mixed with carrier oils, are applied to the body. There is no specific aromatherapy massage, utilizing instead the sweeping and stroking movements of Swedish massage, particularly useful in applying the oils and loosening body tension, and the finger-pressure of shiatsu, used more specifically to relieve pain, tension, fatigue and symptoms of disease. Whilst massage is best undertaken by another person, and the techniques can be learnt from books on aromatherapy, self-massage is also possible. Jackson (1986) devotes a chapter to how this can be achieved, claiming that it is easy, and almost as effective as full-scale treatment.

Massage loosens tight muscles and blocked tissues, focusing on central points in the energy system. As the skin responds, its nerve endings communicate with internal organs, glands, nerves and the circulatory system. The effect can be stimulating or calming, depending on the oils used, and the specific needs of the individual. The massage works on the body and mind simultaneously, calming nerves and stimulating the energy flow, relieving tension and depression, and eliminating toxins, all helping to build healthy tissue.

Aromatherapy uses the essences, or aromatic oils that appear in the various plants. How inhalation of these essences works remains largely unknown. The process of smell is complicated, and whilst theories have been submitted, they remain unproven. Aromas are received by the olfactory receptors in the nose, and from there take a direct route to the limbic area of the brain, which processes smell. The limbic system is the centre of learning, memory and emotions, connected to other parts of the brain which control heart rate, blood-pressure, breathing, reproductive behaviour, memory and reaction to stress. The glands which regulate the release of hormones (and our enjoyment of sex) are also connected to this limbic system.

The inhalation of scent can be achieved indirectly through massage, but also through the use of essential oils in baths. Bathing is a cleansing, relaxing, therapeutic and stimulating activity, particularly when combined with aromatherapy. With the use of steaming and inhalants, it can freshen the skin, and unblock sinuses and congested chests.

Absorption through the skin also raises scientific scepticism, although recent research does indicate that many more substances can pass through the skin than was previously realized. To enable this, the skin has to be cleansed, and made receptive to the oils. Modern diet, make-up, and environmental pollutants have reduced the receptiveness of skin, but the oils are believed to be compatible with the skin's basic structure, and are able to penetrate it, moisturize it, and make it more supple – all processes which stimulate the production of new cells.

Aromatherapy goes beyond the relaxing and stimulating effects of most massage techniques. It is said to have a particular ability to improve sluggish digestion and elimination processes, and to stimulate the lymphatic system, which cleanses and nourishes the blood. Few people realize how vital this system is to health (Chapter 5), and aromatherapy is particularly helpful in liberating blocked lymph nodes, and in improving the function of the lymphatic system.

Each essential oil has different healing properties. When the oils are taken up by the body, some are utilized generally, whilst others are taken up by specific organs. The process through which this is done remains uncertain, but there is no doubt that aromatherapy has considerable value for older people, as it deals with many health problems regularly faced by them, ranging from chronic exhaustion, overweight, skin blemishes, sinus conditions, and stress-related states.

Moreover, the treatments are enjoyable and beneficial, with little danger from toxic side-effects. Like all therapies based on touch, the physical comfort, warmth and security make it an emotionally gratifying way to relax, quite regardless of the aromatic benefits of essential oils. Some of the benefits of these oils have been analysed by Jackson (1986).

- Basil – depression, fainting, mental fatigue, migraine, nausea, nervous tension.
- Cajeput – lung congestion, neuralgia, acne.
- Camomile – skin conditions and inflammations, nervous tension, neuralgia, digestive problems, rheumatism, insomnia.
- Cypress – coughs, rheumatism, flu, wounds, muscle and nerve tension, enlarged veins.
- Geranium –·poor circulation, neuralgia, wounds, burns, mastitis. Also tones the skin.
- Juniper – fatigue, sluggish digestion, water retention, rheumatism, sores.
- Lemon – tonic, antiseptic, diuretic, a preventive for scurvy, age retardant (prevents hardening of body tissues).
- Peppermint – fatigue, indigestion, flatulence, migraine, asthma, bronchitis.
- Pine – infections, water retention, fatigue, rheumatism, gout, flu, bronchitis. Good room disinfectant.
- Sage – fatigue, nervousness, asthma, bronchitis, problems resulting from menopause (contains a natural plant hormone), low blood-pressure. Can be used in a douche.
- Ylang-ylang – high blood-pressure, intestinal infections, impotence. Widely used in fragrances.

Unfortunately, there are problems about the availability and cost of aromatherapy. It is not widely practised in the UK where there is only a handful of aromatherapists, although it is more common in France and on the Continent (Stanway, 1982). Essential oils are also costly, as they are present only in the tiniest amounts in plants, and so have to be painstakingly extracted. They have to be stored in critical conditions to ensure that they retain their potency. Whilst this is undoubtedly an obstacle, the experience of those who experience the pleasure and the health-giving properties of aromatherapy testify to its value.

IONIZATION THERAPY

Air ions were discovered in the nineteenth century. Ionization therapy consists of the use of small, inexpensive electrical machines which give molecules of air a negative electrical charge. Air consists of many gases which are constantly being ionized, or broken down into negatively or positively charged particles. The freshness of air experienced after thunderstorms is the result of the air being negatively charged. In 'fresh' country areas, or seaside air, there are a great number of negatively charged, and fewer positively charged, particles.

Air molecules are positively charged by fumes, dust, smoke and other forms of environmental pollution, including cigarettes. The effect of central heating is to actively create positive ions. The air of industrial, urban areas comprises a large proportion of positively charged ions, which have been proven to be harmful to health (Shreeve, 1986). Ionizers, by increasing the supply of negative ions in the air, have been found to be particularly helpful to patients suffering respiratory disorders, such as colds and influenza, but also asthma and bronchitis. Yet they are known to have many other benefits, perhaps arising from their ability to increase the volume of air taken with each breath, and an increase in the tiny cleansing cells that line the respiratory tract. Stanway (1982) also claims that this can reduce heart rate and blood pressure, and affects the hormone-producing ability of the endocrine glands. They can also be helpful in the treatment of burns and scalds, healing being quickened, without blistering taking place. They are also thought to be helpful with headache and migraine. Generally, ionizers have been found to enhance the sense of energy, vitality and general well-being. They have no side-effects.

OSTEOPATHY

Osteopathy was developed in the USA over 100 years ago by

Andrew Still, a doctor whose personal experience suggested that good health was dependent upon the integrity of the spinal column, and that illness can be explained by structural and mechanical malfunction. The human body was not designed to function in an upright position, so human vertebrae struggle to withstand the constant pressures, and the regular shocks they experience, ultimately leading to the back pain that many people experience. Exercise strengthens the muscles which support the spine, so lack of exercise adds to spinal weakness, and increases the proneness of the modern back to injury and misalignment. Osteopaths also argue that upright posture means that the abdominal organs hang downwards in an unnatural way, causing problems such as hernia, piles, constipation and varicose veins.

Osteopathic success is based on its wider appreciation of the principles of body mechanics, especially in relation to the importance of the spine, and its important association with general health. Treatment is based on the manipulation of the spine, and other joints, seeking to restore them to their normal position and mobility.

Osteopathy is mainly recommended for back pain, either long-standing, or caused by 'ricking' the back by lifting or stooping. Yet as it concentrates on joint manipulation, it can improve the functioning of the entire body. These benefits are believed to arise because the spinal cord, through which the autonomic nervous system is controlled, has direct contact with every part of the body. The central importance of the spine to the skeletal, muscular and nervous systems means that spinal manipulation can benefit ailments not normally associated with back conditions.

Malposition in one part of the body can cause tensions which have to be compensated for elsewhere. Medicine is now recognizing that many illnesses are caused by interference with nerve transmission, due to the pressure, strain or tension on the spinal cord and surrounding tissue, which distorts the information passing to and from the spinal nerves. Muscles then spasm, or become stretched, the nerves become over-sensitive, passing their irritability to the muscles and joints.

Osteopathy has developed the concept of lesions, an area of the body that has become involved in strain, swelling, pain, or the thickening of connective tissue. Most lesions are related to joints, although there need be no identifiable displacement of vertebrae or bone. They are often close to a nerve root, or to an artery in the spinal column, and can adversely affect the mobility of joints, producing tension within the connective tissue, and constricting the blood supply to surrounding tissues and related organs. The close relationship between the nervous system and the circulatory system is of paramount importance to good health. Postural changes affect the spinal vertebrae by compressing the tissue that surrounds nerve roots which can upset this relationship, and produce organ and tissue disease.

By dealing with lesions in specific parts of the body, spinal manipulation can help rebalance the autonomic nervous system that regulates many basic bodily functions, including blood-pressure, heart rate and breathing. Through this process, osteopathy can revitalize problematic pathways, producing dramatic improvements throughout the body, and curing many diseases in internal organs. It can therefore be helpful not only in back pain, but also in the treatment of skin disorders, stomach pain, indigestion, gastric ulcers, bronchitis, asthma and high blood-pressure. Through cranial osteopathy, headache, migraine, epilepsy, deafness and certain eye conditions have also been successfully treated.

Older people suffer from many forms of back pain, ranging from simple backache, rheumatic disorders, lumbago and sciatica. They constitute a major source of unhappiness, reducing the older person's quality of life, and often leading to crippling disablement. The manipulative techniques of osteopathy can be extremely gentle, coaxing the tissues back into place. Sometimes, however, the corrective forces required are greater, and the high-velocity thrust, a short, sharp wrenching movement, is then utilized to release the joint. Even this is usually painless, but it can be extremely successful in reducing, or completely curing, long-standing pain which has withstood the treatment of other medical intervention.

For older people, osteopathy is certainly preferable to increasing doses of pain killers. Pain should be considered a warning of bodily distress, not to be dampened by drugs which can lead to the underlying problems being ignored, which in turn can often lead to even greater damage being caused. The overuse of pain killers, with their increasing toxicity and cumulative dangers of drug side-effects, are particularly hazardous to older people. Osteopathy offers an alternative, which, if more widely utilized, could help prevent this damage, and give pain relief free of side-effects.

Osteopathy is not a self-treatment therapy (although refer to Chaitow, 1990). The manipulation of the spine, and other parts of the body, is a professional task that should not be undertaken by anyone who does not know what he or she is doing. Osteopaths are more common in the USA, where many practitioners have managed to establish themselves as doctors in their own right, and have even received recognition as such from the medical profession. In Britain, osteopathy remains largely unrecognized, and quite independent of conventional medicine.

ACUPUNCTURE

Oriental medicine represents an important element of alternative medicine, with a long and effective history. Its philosophy is very different to that of Western medicine, and has been long derided and castigated by it. Despite this it is becoming increasingly influential. Even medical research is now finding that previously ridiculed ideas have a basis in truth. The preventative aspect of Oriental medicine is particularly noteworthy, perhaps arising from ancient Chinese practice where physicians were paid only when patients were well. When illness struck, payment ceased, providing a powerful incentive for doctors to effect a speedy recovery for their patients (Hope, 1989).

Acupuncture is perhaps the best known form of Oriental medicine. Fulder (1988) summarizes its rise in popularity.

> Twenty years ago acupuncture was assumed to be mere trickery. Fifteen years ago it was somewhat more acceptable provided it was practised on the other side of the planet. Today, it is one of the dominant complementary therapies. The medical profession accepts its effectiveness but restricts its validity to the relief of certain symptoms, in particular pain.

Life is believed to be activated *chi*, the energy, or vital life force, which pervades everything. When *chi* flows freely through the body, health is maintained, but it can be disturbed or interrupted by a variety of factors, some hereditary or constitutional, others the consequence of over-indulgence, emotional trauma, poisoning, climatic change and so on. In understanding the disease, the emphasis is not on germ invasion, but on individual ability to cope with these internal and external factors.

Chi constantly interacts between two poles, the *yin*, the negative, feminine or restraining elements representing coldness, darkness, passivity and inferiority; and the *yang*, the masculine, positive and outgoing elements, representing warmth, light, activity and expressivity. Should either of these aspects become dominant, the harmony of the body is disturbed, and illness results. All forms of Oriental medicine are designed to maintain a balance between these two elements.

A vital feature of Oriental medical philosophy are the 'meridians' – invisible channels that run through the body, connecting with the inner organs, providing the means by which *chi* passes, leading either to health or ill health. There are 12 basic meridians related to the major organs or functions to which they are associated. Six are predominantly *yin*: heart, heart protector, spleen, lungs, kidney and liver: and six predominantly *yang*: small intestine, triple heater, colon, stomach, bladder and gall-bladder (Fulder, 1988).

These have never been anatomically verified, and so have been dismissed. However, recent research has begun to discover a basis in science for them. Perhaps this indicates that man's best means of progress is through intuition rather than science. Science will catch up eventually.

Acupuncture involves the insertion of needles into the skin at specific points for the purpose of treating various disorders by stimulating *chi*. Acupuncture points may bear little relationship to the area for which treatment is sought, but are chosen along the meridians which correspond to the different organs of the body. The needles vary in thickness, penetrate to varying depths, and can be inserted for varying amounts of time. They can be rotated clockwise, or pumped, to stimulate energy flow. Moxibustion consists of placing a cone of moxa (*artemisia vulgaris*) over the selected acupuncture point and lighting it.

Acupuncture also recognizes 12 different pulses, six in each wrist, and each corresponding to one of the meridians. By feeling these pulses, experienced practitioners are able to diagnose any imbalances in the flow of *chi* which might be causing illness, and thereby determine the treatment which is required.

Acupuncture is capable of curing most conditions, and in preventing the establishment or spread of most diseases, but it is best known for its ability to relieve pain, even long-standing and intractable pain. It has been found that acupuncture triggers the release of pituitary endorphins, which are passed to the spinal cord from where they can exert an opiate-like effect on the perception of pain. Indeed, acupuncture is used in China as a form of analgesia in major surgical operations, with patients remaining fully conscious, but in no apparent discomfort, or post-operation distress.

As pain is a major problem for many older people, the potential value of acupuncture is clear. It has been found that most people who consult acupuncturists are the 'hopeless cases', pronounced incurable by allopathic medicine; yet acupuncture was found to lead to improved health for 70% of them (Stanway, 1982). Whilst this indicates the value of acupuncture, it is probably a misuse of it. Most practitioners feel that acupuncture is best used as a means of maintaining, rather than rehabilitating, health.

Acupuncture is not a self-help therapy; it has to be applied by trained therapists. However, shiatsu and acupressure work on the same principle as acupuncture, with the fingers taking the place of needles.

SHIATSU AND ACUPRESSURE

Shiatsu and acupressure substitute finger pressure for needles along the same meridian points as acupunture. There are no essential differences between the two techniques. Pressure is applied generally over the entire body, but with particular attention being paid to the points on the meridians. The objective is to search for painful, hot or knotted areas, to which specific attention is given. When a 'problem' area is found, sufficient pressure is applied to act deeply, perhaps causing the sensation of discomfort, but stopping short of being painful. The degree and type of pressure depends upon many factors, and is usually repeated three or four times, each for several seconds.

Shiatsu and acupressure can relieve many kinds of chronic aches and pains. They are particularly helpful in treating stress disorders, such as migraine headaches, and rheumatic and circulatory disorders. They are also helpful with depression, constipation, insomnia and diarrhoea. They are said to have either a calming or stimulating effect (some claim that they have an effect on sexual functioning), the particular effect depending on the needs of the individual.

As neither equipment or oils are used, they are excellent self-help techniques, and methods of first aid. Shiatsu is widely used for this purpose in Japan, often being mutually applied between family members. There are few practitioners available, but there are a number of books providing instructions for self-treatment, for example, Kenyon (1987). They are also entirely safe techniques, as it is difficult to use too much pressure on your own body and, unlike needles, there is more leeway in the areas that need to be stimulated.

REFLEXOLOGY

Reflexology is another technique acting upon the life-force flowing through the meridians, and is based on a system of foot massage discovered by Dr W. Fitzgerald in the 1920s, but developed from forms of therapy used in China and India over 5000 years ago.

151

Reflexologists claim that the entire body is mirrored in the feet. Thus, through foot massage, health benefits can arise in parts of the body quite removed from the foot, primarily by stimulating the healing forces inherent within the body, and increasing the body's ability to heal itself. This should not be a surprise, for as Stanway (1982) states, it is well known that the internal organs are represented on the surface of the body by areas of skin that share the same nerve supplies as these organs. He gives an example of conditions affecting the diaphragm, which can often present as pain in the shoulder tip, simply because both share the same nerve supply. Experiments on animals have indicated that by stimulating the skin surface representing an organ, physiological effects can be produced in the related organ.

The body is divided into 'zones' of energy that form the basis for the prevention and treatment of illness. Ten channels have been identified, each beginning in an area of the foot, travelling from there throughout the entire body. Each channel relates to the organs that belong to that particular zone.

Reflexologists are able to detect blocked channels, and identify the organs, or related parts of the body, that are not functioning properly. These 'blocks' can be located by special massage techniques. The terminals in each reflex in each foot are explored and analysed by applying pressure at certain points, rotating the toes, moving the foot up and down, rubbing the skin or simply sensing with the finger-tips. Problem areas are located when a tenderness is found in a particular part of the foot. These can feel like small granular lumps under the skin, crystalline deposits on the nerve endings which are the cause of blockages. Gentle massage disperses these granules, which are absorbed by the circulatory system, and excreted from the body.

Reflexology is comprehensive in its impact on health. It can treat all conditions, although it will not cure infectious conditions, and it will not deal with structural problems. In a full treatment, all the parts (or reflexes) of both feet are massaged, improving the circulation of blood to the corresponding part of the body, removing waste deposits and congestion, assisting glandular function, reducing nervous tensions in problem areas, and relaxing the whole body, including the mind. It restores the correct flow of energy throughout the body, and adjusts the imbalances that cause ill health.

Reflexology is effective in treating many ailments suffered by older people. It is particularly effective in relieving tension, stiffness and pain. Many people find it helpful in dispelling symptoms of stress, helping relaxation and sleep, and producing a sense of revitalization and well being. It is also good for unblocking sinuses, relieving headaches and migraine, and assisting liver, kidney and pancreas function. It is effective with constipation, and can also benefit people suffering from arthritis, asthma, circulatory problems, diabetes, epilepsy, glandular disease and hypertension.

Reflexology is a painless alternative to strong drug treatment, entirely free of side-effects, although after treatment minor illness can develop, this being interpreted as the body eliminating toxic material. It is a method that ideally lends itself to self-help.

ALTERNATIVE MEDICINE: ITS AVAILABILITY AND COST

In 1981, the *Threshold Survey* attempted to estimate the number of alternative therapists in the UK (Fulder, 1988). It found that there were over 11 000 therapists belonging to professional bodies practising during that year. The figures in Table 9.1 were given to indicate the availability of practitioners in the therapies outlined in this chapter.

Table 9.1 Availability of alternative medicine practitioners

Therapy	Medically qualified	In a professional association	Not in a professional association	Total
Acupuncture	160	548	250	958
Alexander technique	5	170	50	225
Herbalism	10	228	200	438
Homeopathy	425	41	230	696
Naturopathy	5	204	200	409
Osteopathy	212	777	150	1139

Most alternative therapists are private practitioners who charge a fee for consultations. These fees are usually not high, and certainly considerably cheaper than consulting an allopathic specialist privately. They are in the region of about £15 to £25 per single session. The first session is often a double session, when the individual is asked to give a full personal history, enabling the therapist to build a complete, or holistic, picture of the individual.

Homeopathic and herbal remedies are also inexpensive. Indeed, the cost for a small bottle of a single remedy is now less than the cost of a National Health prescription. However, as pensioners do not pay prescriptions, remedies do imply a cost. Aromatherapy oils are more expensive.

153

However, many people after years of ineffective treatment, are prepared to pay for an alternative which can provide good results, in which they have confidence, and they know to be safe.

Alternative medicine is often used as a last, rather than a first, resort in the event of illness, something to be tried when all else, including allopathic treatment, has failed. The reverse might be more sensible and appropriate, particularly as many therapies are particularly focused on preventative, rather than curative, intervention.

10

Treating the illnesses of old age

How should older people deal with illness? To whom should they turn? What can be done to maintain health, and what do the various forms of treatment offer? The overall aim for older people should be to minimize the encroachment that illness has on activity and enjoyment. The fact that heart disease may be more responsive to relaxation than tablets, that ulcers can be cured by diet, and that most illnesses can be prevented by simple lifestyle changes is becoming increasingly clear, whilst at the same time, the failure of allopathic medicine becomes more widely appreciated.

The complexity of advice and the plethora of medical experts available for consultation can be confusing, and often leads to people seeking one, single 'expert' with all the answers. It is important to resist such confusion, and avoid reliance on one opinion. The diversity of medical advice results from a single cause; no one is certain, no single approach has all the answers. Yet each approach has something to offer. The choice, however complex it might appear, is for individuals to make on the basis of their own preferences.

This chapter considers several broad groups of illnesses, with the emphasis placed on their prevention rather than treatment, and self-help rather than professional involvement. *What follows does not represent medical advice, only general guidance on where to look for that advice, and the wide variety of sources from which help can be obtained.*

The contribution of allopathic medicine is examined in order to redress the balance of medical information and power, questioning whether it should be used as our first resort, and indicating some reasons for looking elsewhere for the maintenance and restoration of health. Moreover, by giving details of the side-effects of many drugs, it can also indicate where current medication is leading to iatrogenic health problems.

Alternative medical therapies, in comparison to the complexity of allopathic philosophy, intimate that all illness is traceable to a single overall cause, an inner disharmony with which the body cannot cope, and that the basis for this disharmony is usually nutritional, emotional or environmental. Such an interpretation avoids the need to minutely define and categorize illness, although it also means that the 'solutions' offered can appear repetitious. This merely highlights the relative simplicity of good health, as an entity that lays within the reach of each individual, and one that offers freedom from medicalization.

CARDIOVASCULAR AILMENTS

The heart has an enormous workload, beating daily around 100 000 times and pumping 7 tons of blood around the body. The blood vessels, consisting of 60 000 miles of arteries and veins, have to expand and contract alongside the heart. Fortunately, the heart is an extremely strong muscle, and the circulatory system very tough. When problems arise, they are usually the result of long-standing abuse rather than inherent weakness, or the ravages of the ageing process. Until this century, heart disease was not a major concern; indeed, angina pectoris was not known until 1772, and before the 1920s coronary heart disease was regarded as an uncommon disease (Ashton and Davies, 1986). Now it has become a major cause of death, even for apparently fit and healthy people.

Heart disease remains virtually absent in underdeveloped countries. Even in Japan, where there is less consumption of fatty foods and sugar, the incidence of heart disease is low. However, Japanese people living in the USA quickly become as vulnerble as US citizens. This indicates that lifestyle abuses the modern heart, and heart disease can be avoided by attention to these factors.

Arteriosclerosis and atherosclerosis The former is the hardening or gradual loss of elasticity in the walls of arteries; *atherosclerosis* is where cholesterol and other fats are deposited in the inner linings of arteries. Both conditions narrow the arteries, reduce blood flow, weaken circulation, raise blood-pressure, and lead to the degeneration of some internal organs. Together, they form the major cause of heart disease, and are often considered to be age related as they are found more commonly in older than younger people. However, they probably do not result from normal ageing.

156

Hypertension This is consistently high blood-pressure caused by the thickening of the blood. Early indications of hypertension include dizziness, headaches, agitation and nosebleeds. Hypertension places the heart, arteries and other organs under stress, leading to impaired kidney function, defective metabolism, increased toxaemia, arteriosclerosis, susceptibility to heart failure and strokes.

Angina pectoris This is severe pain in the centre of the chest, often following simple exertion or emotional stress, caused by insufficient blood reaching the heart, and is often the result of arteriosclerosis. It is a warning of more serious coronary heart disease.

Coronary heart attacks or thromboses These are caused by the obstruction of coronary vessels, usually by blood clots, or thromboses, forming on the walls of coated arteries. The reduced supply of blood to the heart muscle eventually causes a heart attack. Although the condition now affects all age-groups, the furring up of arteries over the years increases the risk for older people.

Strokes Although not a cardiovascular ailment, strokes involve the destruction of brain cells brought about when the brain is starved of blood by a clot, or damaged by haemorrhage; both are associated with hypertension. The area of brain affected ceases to operate, bringing sudden, total or partial unconsciousness, but affecting the individual in ways specific to the part of the brain destroyed. It is a crippling, degenerative ailment, often leaving the individual paralysed down one side, and becomes increasingly common with ageing people, particularly in active people after retirement. The apparent suddenness of strokes suggest that they occur by chance or misfortune. This is not so; many years of neglect prepare the individual for heart disease of all types. Before strokes occur, individuals usually manifest signs of hypertension, arteriosclerosis and chronic kidney dysfunction.

Allopathic treatment

There are now many tests available for measuring blood-pressure and blood cholesterol levels. If heart disease is discovered sufficiently early, and the individual reacts positively through dietary modification and increased exercise, it can be treated without drug or surgical intervention. Despite this, the main response to heart disease

157

is drug treatment. Indeed, there is a tendency to prescribe medication for even mild blood-pressure.

The main drugs are antiarrhythmics, for heart rhythm abnormalities, which relax the heart muscle; anticoagulants, which stop the formation of blood clots; antihypertensives, which reduce blood-pressure; calcium antagonists, used for angina pain; vasodilators, which increase the size of blood vessels and reduce blood-pressure; diuretics, which reduce excess liquid and salt in the body and reduce blood-pressure; and beta blockers, used to block the action of adrenaline in the heart.

These all offer temporary amelioration rather than cure for heart disease. There is little evidence that they improve general health, and no indication that they extend, or improve, quality of life to any significant degree. Once started, they are often taken permanently, as cessation usually means that benefits disappear immediately. They cause many side-effects: antiarrhythmics cause dizziness and vision problems; anticoagulants cause bleeding and bruising; antihypertensives cause constipation, headaches, diarrhoea and dizziness; beta blockers cause dizziness, constipation and diarrhoea, low blood-pressure and drowsiness; diuretics cause headaches, drowsiness and nausea; vasodilators cause palpitations and nausea. They can all cause vitamin and mineral deficiencies, leading to fatigue, sleeping difficulties, loss of appetite, impotence, depression and confusion.

This is by no means a comprehensive list of side-effects, and older people can suffer more severely owing to the body metabolizing and eliminating drugs more slowly. They can be particularly dangerous if the individual already suffers from asthma, diabetes, kidney and other disorders.

In major heart disease, special intensive care units are available, although the benefit of these expensive units is being questioned, with evidence that patient survival after heart attacks might be slightly better if they remain at home (Inglis and West, 1983). Surgical treatment also fails to deal with the underlying cause of heart disease. The fitting of electronic pacemakers controls irregular heartbeat, and by-pass surgery replaces blocked blood vessels with portions of vein removed from elsewhere in the body. These are often effective, but only if the individual subsequently alters his or her lifestyle to avoid reoccurrence. Heart transplantation is increasing, despite little evidence that it confers longer life, or justifies the enormous expense in time and resources.

Prevention

Those people who survive coronary heart disease, and have sufficient determination to change their lifestyle, can continue to live abundantly; but not in the same way. Conversely, without changing the factors which increase vulnerability to heart disease, no medicine can maintain health. For most people, avoidance of and recovery from heart disease requires a change in lifestyle, with diet, exercise and stress being the primary features of both prevention and cure, along with obesity, personality factors and smoking.

A cleansing diet is required that reduces the furring-up of arteries, and lowers blood cholesterol and high blood-pressure. It is the consumption of saturated fats that increases blood cholesterol levels, and accelerates the narrowing of coronary arteries, resulting in an unhealthy bloodstream which produces clotting. Obesity is a known cause of high blood-pressure and heart disease. Reducing the consumption of fat is vital, best achieved by avoiding meat, eggs and dairy products.

These can be replaced with natural foods such as nuts, seeds, soya beans, and fresh fruit and vegetables. Fresh garlic and fish, such as salmon, tuna, mackerel and herrings, are beneficial because they are known to prevent the formation of blood clots. Dietary fibre is also important, as this assists the body in dealing with cholesterol.

Salt and food additives are also implicated in raising blood-pressure. The per capita consumption of salt in the UK is about 25 times greater than required, salt being found in all canned food, sauces, processed meat and cheese. Salt consumption should be reduced drastically, particularly with people already suffering from heart disease.

Exercise is a vital factor in strengthening the cardiovascular system. It is common for heart disease patients to believe that exercise is harmful, even dangerous to health. The reality is that exercise becomes more important both as a preventative and curative measure. Inadequate exercise is characteristic of most people with heart disease, with continuing inactivity further perpetuating problems. Even after coronary heart disease, the individual can exercise gently, although this should not be pursued beyond the point that chest pain develops. Regular exercise stabilizes blood-pressure, keeps the blood supply in good condition, improves the oxygen-carrying properties of the blood, produces additional 'high-density lipoproteins', which remove silt deposits from arteries, and can contribute to the eventual recovery of the circulatory system. It is also known that exercise can stimulate the development of new blood vessels to the heart. How this is done is uncertain, but when exercise increases the demand for blood, nature would appear to increase both the number and size of vessels in order to meet the demand (Cailliet and Gross, 1987).

Emotional stress is another important factor in heart disease. Tense posture and tight muscles increase resistance to blood circulation, particularly with inactive people, and in situations like driving, where exercise is not possible. How stress is removed is dependent upon its individual source. The ability to relax, to spend time following enjoyable pursuits, to maintain emotional control, and exercise regularly, and the ability to sleep soundly, are all vital.

Popular means of stress reduction are harmful. The nicotine inhaled by smoking accelerates the hardening of arteries, reduces the amount of oxygen available to the heart, encourages the formation of blood clotting, and stimulates the production of adrenalin, which makes the heart beat harder and faster. Stimulants, such as tea and coffee, are also implicated in heart disease, with caffeine increasing blood cholesterol and raising blood-pressure. Camomile tea is a healthier alternative, having a calming effect on the central nervous system, helping to relieve tension, confusion and muscle cramp. Indeed, several herbal teas are helpful soothers, including sage, rosemary, hops, valerian, parsley, fenugreek and hawthorn.

Alternative medicine

Most alternative therapies regard dietary and lifestyle changes as the key to a sound, healthy heart. Their main response is to correct the underlying factors leading to heart disease, not to tackle the disease process itself. Most resist direct treatment, instead relying upon reforming lifestyle factors.

After serious heart disease, naturopaths usually recommend complete rest, a supervised fast, with the individual being kept calm and warm. Following this, the individual is encouraged to maintain a strict dietary regime, involving wholefoods, without saturated fats; drinking and smoking is banned, and exercise is encouraged; stress is best dealt with through relaxation.

Herbal medicine can provide many remedies which improve circulation, such as yarrow, elderflower, hyssop and buckwheat. Calming remedies, like valerian, have been used for centuries for stress-related heart problems, as have rosemary, lavender and lady's slipper. The World Health Organization has studied many traditional herbs, used for centuries for heart disease, and several, including valerian, garlic, geranium, mistletoe, olive and hawthorn have been validated (Hoffman, 1990). Other treatments, such as the use of foot and hand baths, are also recommended.

Aromatherapy uses several essences, including garlic, lavender and ylang-ylang; and, for stroke victims, massaging the spinal column, and the paralysed parts can be helpful.

Homeopathy can provide many remedies which work by purifying the blood, and supporting the work of the kidneys, liver and skin in cleansing the body of toxins. Arnica, aconite and baryta carb is used for stroke victims; nux vomica, arsenicum, digitalis and lachesis for heart disease; cactus for angina; and nat mur and argentum nit for hypertension. It should be stressed, however, that remedies are prescribed for individuals, not for generalized conditions.

Massage therapies can be useful, particularly with stroke victims. Reflexology works on the reflexes which relate to the solar plexus, heart, lungs and bronchial tubes. Osteopathy can aid the rehabilitation of stroke victims.

Acupuncture has been shown to produce a marked increase in the functional ability and efficiency of heart muscles (Shreeve, 1986), reducing blood-pressure, improving poor circulation and increasing the supply of blood to the brain. It has been effective in the treatment of stroke victims when used soon after the attack.

Relaxation therapies are important for stress related conditions, particularly with people with 'Type A' personality. Yoga helps in bringing both serenity and calm, and also through its basic exercises and positions. The latter can be particularly helpful for stroke victims in recovering the use of their limbs.

DIGESTIVE AILMENTS

The body requires a constant supply of energy, which comes mainly from food, and which is broken down by the digestive system into nutrients the body can use. These food nutrients are eventually absorbed into the blood stream, which carries them to the cells throughout the body. The digestive system begins at the mouth, includes the pharynx, oesophagus, stomach, colon, the small and large intestine, and the rectum, and works closely with the pancreas, liver and gall-bladder.

Digestive problems have been called the 'diseases of civilization' as they are pandemic in the industrialized world. The reason is modern diet, with the consumption of processed and refined foods, high in animal fats and sugar, and devoid of fibre, usually being consumed in quantities the body cannot handle. The bowel needs to be regularly evacuated to prevent poisonous wastes from building up, but when too much fat, and too little fibrous food is eaten, decaying faeces can remain for long periods, congesting the entire digestive system.

Constipation This is the incomplete or infrequent action of the bowels, with the consequent filling of the rectum with hard faeces, producing considerable pain and discomfort for many older people. Constipation can ultimately lead to more serious conditons, such as piles, varicose veins and, it has been suggested, could even result in bowel cancer.

Colitis This is the inflammation of the colon, caused by its toxic contents. Food, particularly meat, putrefies in the colon, and this toxic material can eventually damage the mucous membrane, in time leading to diverticulitis and cancer.

Diverticulitis Diverticula are tiny balloons of intestinal lining which break through the muscular wall of the intestine, usually in the colon. Common symptoms are anal bleeding, constipation, diarrhoea and lower, left-sided abdominal pain. Intestinal obstruction or abscesses may develop.

Gastric and duodenal ulcers, and ulcerative colitis These are persistent sores, or loss of mucous membrane, caused by digestive juices, which normally function by breaking down food passing through the stomach, turning their attention instead to the linings of the stomach walls. Ulcerative conditions, common with older people, are classified according to the part of the digestive system where they occur.

Haemorrhoids Commonly known as piles, these are a painful varicose condition of the veins at the lower end of the rectum, and are associated with obesity and constipation.

Gallstones The gall-bladder acts as a reservoir for bile, a digestive fluid secreted by the liver. Gallstones are hard, insoluble concretions, composed of bile pigments, cholesterol and calcium salts, which form in the gall-bladder with painful consequences. Symptoms are indigestion, nausea, biliousness, and upper-right abdominal pain. They are associated with older people, particularly those with high levels of cholesterol in their blood.

Allopathic treatment

The direct connection between digestive problems and diet is clear, with food passing through the stomach, intestines and bowels. Despite this, medical practice continues to treat these conditions with drugs, indicating that medication is considered more effective than dietary change. Dietary changes are recommended, although advice often concentrates on easing the painfulness of digestion, rather than helping the condition directly.

This is best demonstrated by responses to constipation, perhaps the earliest sign of digestive problems. Although it is known that constipation is caused largely by an inadequate intake of dietary fibre, it is still treated primarily by the prescription of laxatives. Whilst these are easy to use, they have little long-term effectiveness, and harmful side-effects in causing weakness of intestinal muscles, sometimes to the point that normal defecation ceases.

Antacids relieve pain by neutralizing acid in the stomach, and are used to treat indigestion, and ulcer pain. They are widely used, both by prescription and retail sale. Their side-effects range from appetite loss, blurred vision, palpitations and swollen ankles.

Anticholinergic and antispasmodic drugs reduce acid production, and the spasms which can occur in the stomach and intestines. They are also used in the treatment of ulcers. They can cause constipation, headache, irregular heartbeat, nausea, visual problems and, in older people, confusion.

Antidiarrhoeal drugs seek to help diarrhoea and colitis by reducing the intestinal tract's muscle activity. They are not usually prescribed for very old people as they can cause incontinence, abdominal pain, diarrhoea and stool impaction; they can also cause depression, drowsiness, headaches, insomnia and loss of appetite.

Modern ulcer-healing drugs, such as cimetidine, revolutionized ulcer treatment, and were initially acclaimed as a medical breakthrough as they relieve ulcer pain quickly, and stop internal bleeding. However, the main problem with all these drugs is the high rate of relapse after treatment is discontinued. But they are now also known to produce nitrosamines, which cause stomach cancer, and are associated with impotence, diarrhoea, dizziness, liver disorders, muscle pain and tiredness; with older people they can cause confusion and disorientation.

If drug action is not effective, surgery is often used. Gallstones are often removed by surgery and, in severe conditions, the gallbladder itself can be removed. The removal of damaged parts of the colon is sometimes the treatment for colitis.

Many stomach disorders are themselves provoked by medication, such as tranquillizers, antidepressants, analgesics and antacids, taken orally for other medical conditions. Overall, it would seem best to discard pills, which only deal with symptoms, and take some difficult dietary decisions.

Prevention

Good diet is vital in preventing digestive orders, with wholefood, fresh fruit and vegetables being particularly important. A high-fibre diet is needed to propel stomach contents efficiently through the digestive system. The avoidance of sweet foods is also important, as Shakespeare noted when he commented, 'things sweet to taste prove in digestion sour'. More recently, it has been suggested that certain food combinations are unhelpful, with the Hay Diet, for example, suggesting that it is helpful to separate the eating of protein, fruit and carbohydrates.

Insufficient fluid intake can result in constipation, and there is evidence to suggest that alcohol, Indian teas and coffee should be avoided. In contrast, dandelion, fennel and camomile teas can aid digestion, whilst flax and liquorice can assist bowel evacuation.

Lack of exercise, so often associated with old age, can lead to constipation and subsequent digestive problems. Exercise is an excellent way of encouraging bowel movement, and preventing further problems with digestion in old age.

Alternative therapies

Most alternative practitioners believe that diet should be the focus of treatment, although they also recognize the benefits of exercise, stress and other factors. When illness strikes, treatment aims to support liver and kidney function in order to encourage their detoxifying and regulating effects on health.

Naturopathy has a particular role with digestive problems, as it concentrates upon diet to the exclusion of all other forms of treatment. Naturopaths seek to cleanse the stomach, first by fasting, and then by strict dietary control which avoids meat, fish, hard cheese, dairy products and eggs, recommending instead a vegetarian diet, with fresh fruit, especially grapefruit and pears, and fresh vegetables.

There are large numbers of herbal remedies for stomach disorders, for which they are ideally suited, and have a long tradition. These include aloe vera, balmony, barberry, black root, comfrey, dandelion, figwort, flax seed, marshmallow, rhubarb, sage, senna, vervain, wahoo, wild yam and yellow dock (Hoffman, 1983). Many are used to treat minor stomach upsets, some for constipation, and others for ulcers. Camomile is worth special mention, as it is ideally suited for digestive problems, has been used since ancient times, and is readily available in the form of tea. Aromatherapy, likewise, can offer many helpful remedies for digestive conditions.

Homeopathy offers remedies which seek to balance the natural metabolic process, and which are also used for specific ailments. Haemorrhoids are treated with calc fluor, ignatia, nux vomica; for diverticulitis, lycopodium and ipecacuanha; for colitis, argentum nit and arsenicum album; for ulcers, ornithogalum; with chelidonium being used for gallstones (Shreeve, 1986). Homeopathy can also help with remedies for emotional factors, which unbalance the natural rhythm of digesting and assimilating food, and the excretion of waste materials.

Oriental therapies utilize the meridians associated with the stomach and large intestine. Acupuncture has been shown to reduce stomach acidity, discharge gallstones, and can assist with colitis, diverticulitis and ulcers.

Exercise therapies are important, particularly for diverticulitis, and relaxation therapies for stress-related conditions, particularly ulcers. Yoga is recommended on both counts. And whilst digestive disorders are not their usual speciality, osteopathy can assist with digestive problems, as the cause of digestive problems is often related to spinal defects.

RESPIRATORY AILMENTS

The respiratory system begins with the nose, which takes air via the larynx and trachea to the lungs. Oxygen is essential for the release of energy which supports the continuation of life. The lungs execute the vital task of extracting oxygen from the air, reoxygenating the blood, and discharging from the body poisonous waste products, principally carbon dioxide and water.

Bronchitis This is the inflammation and congestion of the bronchial tubes, which blocks the free flow of air to the lungs. Its acute form often develops after influenza, measles, and other upper respiratory conditions (naturopaths would claim that bronchitis arises from the suppression of these conditions), inducing malaise, muscle pain, sore throat and fever. It can lead to emphysema and pneumonia. Chronic bronchitis is common amongst older people, particularly those with a history of smoking, or working and living in polluted industrial atmospheres.

Emphysema This is a chronic condition in which the lungs do not expand and contract in the normal way, but remain in a state of constant inflation. It is associated with a build-up of heavy phlegm, and is common amongst long-term, heavy smokers.

Asthma This is a condition arising from the bronchi of the lungs contracting in spasm, narrowing the airways, and causing shortness of breath, wheezing, choking and suffocation. It is often caused by allergy in younger people, but can be brought on by infections, stress or psychological upsets (or attempts to suppress the symptoms of such conditions).

Allopathic treatment

Antihistamines work by blocking the action of histamine, a natural body chemical, released in response to injury, allergy or irritation, leading to hay fever, nasal congestion and related symptoms. Their side-effects include constipation, diarrhoea, dizziness and depression, whilst with older people they are associated with urinary problems, confusion and extreme drowsiness.

Antibiotics are often prescribed for bronchitis, when considered to be caused by bacterial infection. They can prove effective, but there is increasing recognition of the iatrogenic problems associated with their overuse.

Asthma is usually treated using inhalers, or bronchodilators, initially introduced as an instant, miracle cure for asthma attacks. Unfortunately, when overused they were found to damage the heart, and tripled the death rate. Whilst their lethal impact has been modified, it is also suspected that over-reliance on inhalers can lead to the reinforcement of faulty breathing patterns, which can compound long-term problems.

Prevention

The first essential is to stop smoking, which is a direct and deliberate assault on the lungs, and to inhale the cleanest possible air. Unfortunately, air pollution is hard to avoid, and whilst the respiratory system is usually able to cope, heavily polluted air increases the impurities taken directly into the lungs, creating catarrhal congestion which accumulates until respiratory illness develops. This is exacerbated for individuals who live or work in cold, damp, dusty, smoky or foggy atmospheres.

Correct breathing is important. If air is taken through the mouth, air filtration depends solely upon hair-like projections on the internal lining of the trachea, which deal with foreign material, but if air is taken correctly through the nose, similar hairs in the nostrils act as preliminary filters. Associated with correct breathing is the importance of exercise, which has direct effects on maintaining the efficiency of the respiratory system.

Food sensitivity, and contact with common domestic chemicals, have received increasing recognition, particularly in asthma which is known to be closely linked to allergy. A diet which avoids additives, refined and processed foods, tea, coffee and alcohol, and which instead concentrates on wholefoods, is usually recommended. Exclusion diets are sometimes necessary, with particular attention being paid to wheat, milk and dairy products. Vitamin C is a natural antihistamine, and the anti-infective qualities of garlic is also increasingly recognized.

Emotional factors can also lower general resistance, particularly in asthma, because respiratory changes are often associated with fear.

Alternative therapies

Alternative medicine does not blame viruses as the cause of ailments, and agrees that suppressing the symptoms of respiratory ailments is counter-productive. There is growing awareness that colds and influenza should be allowed to take their normal course, as these are the body's attempt to throw off toxicity within the body, and suppression ultimately produces more serious problems. Instead, alternative therapies focus on the root of the problem, which concerns the body's ability to deal with the quality of air that we breath. Ionizers, placed in bedrooms and living areas, are helpful in filtering air, reducing air pollution, assisting breathing, and can be recommended.

167

Naturopathy encourages fasts, followed by a diet of raw vegetables, increased drinking of fruit juices, and thereafter the avoidance of rich food, which aids the formation of mucus. There are innumerable herbal remedies, perhaps best used for the prevention of respiratory disorders. Drinking herb teas, including aniseed, dill, camomile, hops, eucalyptus and liquorice, can help to settle the respiratory tract, calm the nerves, and induce restful sleep. Similarly, there are a variety of homeopathic remedies which support the body's own resistance to respiratory ailments, particularly bryonia and ipecacuanha.

Psychological aspects of respiratory disorders, especially stress, point to the value of relaxation techniques, such as yoga, and aromatherapy, both particularly helpful in preventing and treating respiratory disorders. Bad posture and incorrect breathing are often implicated in respiratory disorders, so the Alexander principle and yoga can be helpful, as can manipulative techniques, such as reflexology and shiatsu. Acupuncture has also demonstrated its effectiveness with respiratory ailments.

PAIN

The sensation of pain is an important warning that the body is experiencing some form of physical disorders that requires investigation. Pain occurs in the bones, muscles, connective tissues, and the articulated joints, which enable movement. The joints are particularly vulnerable, for in order to fulfil the heavy mechanical work expected of them, they require lubrication by synovial fluid produced by the body, and transported via the blood. If joints receive insufficient lubrication, pain develops which restricts mobility, with immobility causing stiffness, increased pain, and a further reduction in mobility. This is a common sequence with older people.

Osteoarthritis This is a degenerative condition attacking the cartilage of weight-bearing joints (the hips, knees and shoulders particularly), aggravated by an impaired blood supply, previous injury and obesity. Arthritis was once considered a disease of older people, but young children, even infants, are now found to suffer from it. Arthritis does not kill, but is a disabling condition which makes life unpleasant and painful. It has more impact on the quality of life than many other, more lethal, diseases.

Rheumatoid arthritis (rheumatism) This is a chronic inflammation of the joints, especially the fingers, wrists, hands, vertebrae, ankles and elbows, often causing bone deformity. The condition often follows a number of infections, such as rubella and tuberculosis, and is a common feature of fevers. Alternative practitioners would suggest that it arises from the suppression of symptoms of these illnesses. The disease usually affects older people, and can be progressively incapacitating, affecting, in turn, the skin, eyes, kidneys, heart, lungs and blood.

Bone, like any other tissue of the body, is dynamic, and depending on the inner health of the body, bone is either being formed or broken down. The bones of older people can become thinner and more fragile, giving rise to other diseases.

Osteoporosis This is a change in the texture of bones caused by a loss of calcium which makes them brittle, and represents the major single cause of fractures in older people.

Osteomalacia This is a disease characterized by painful softening of the bone due to vitamin D and calcium deficiency. The loss of protein and calcium, essential components of bone formation and maintenance, is often incorrectly associated with ageing, and a decline in bodily vigour. It is particularly associated with post-menopausal women, when hormonal changes, along with changes in activity and diet (and the surgical removal of ovaries), also cause a loss of calcium. The conditions can lead to tiredness, weakness, pain in the back, trunk and limbs, and eventually physical deformity.

It is important to attribute pain to disease rather than age, for this constitutes the basis of the ageist neglect that older people with painful ailments have been subjected to. The essential argument about pain is that it has a medical cause, and is not the natural penalty of age. Pain can be treated, arrested or even cured by a variety of medical treatments.

Allopathic treatment

Pain, particularly arthritic pain, is a common problem for which allopathic medicine offers only pain-killers, palliatives which fail to address causation, and make no pretence at effecting cure. Fast pain relief is possible, but relief is temporary, and the drugs cause considerable side-effects. Arthritis pain relieved by drugs does not treat the toxicity which is its cause; indeed, it adds to it. The suppression of pain leads ultimately to more pain, stronger pain-killers, more assaults on body tissue and, ultimately, to immobility and joint replacement.

Analgesics, such as aspirin, are widely used to suppress pain. Its most well-known side-effect is to cause stomach disorders, including intestinal bleeding; but it can also lead to deafness, heartburn, blood disorders, bronchial problems, diarrhoea and constipation, dizziness, drowsiness and vision problems. Drugs based on paracetamol cause fatigue and weakness, drowsiness, dizziness, nausea, light-headedness, low blood-pressure, constipation and depression, and, in older people, have been associated with kidney, liver and pancreas problems. Corticosteroids, heralded as a wonder drug for suppressing inflammation, have been found to suppress the body's immune defence against infection, can raise blood-pressure, increase weight, and can cause osteoporosis, ulcers, cataracts, diabetes, insomnia and severe depression. Opren, marketed as a wonder drug suitable for older people, was withdrawn when it caused numerous fatalities.

Steroidal medication, also used for asthma, is known to aggravate the loss of calcium, and can lead to the development of osteoporosis. The allopathic treatment for these conditions in post-menopausal women is hormone replacement thereapy. Even this treatment is now implicated with an increased risk of cancer.

Non-steroidal anti-inflammatory drugs can cause diarrhoea, digestive problems, intestinal bleeding, headache, nausea, blood disorders, chest pain, hearing and vision disorders, drowsiness, light-headedness, swelling legs, hands and feet, ulcers, and high blood-pressure; they are widely used for older people, making the aged particularly susceptible to constipation, reduced alertness, and kidney disease.

Traction, corsets and plaster casts and, ultimately, the replacement of diseased joints, is the surgical response at the chronic end of pain.

Prevention

There is little archaeological evidence to suggest that these conditions existed before the seventeenth century to anywhere near the extent that they do now, indicating that they, like heart disease, are associated with modern lifestyle, and the result of internal toxicity arising from the modern diet. The refined sugar, white flour products, and fat meats, all introduce toxicity to the body more quickly than it can be eliminated, particularly when modern food refining and over-cooking also destroys the alkaline mineral salts essential in neutralizing acidity (Hills, 1985). The blood becomes increasingly toxic, with acid deposits leading to pain and chronic illness in the joints, bones and muscles.

Pain must be treated seriously. Diet is crucial in reversing the process of increasing pain and declining mobility. Some cases of arthritis respond to a gluten-free diet, which omits wheat, rye, oats and barley. Others have found that foods, such as potatoes, peppers, chilli, paprika, pimento, aubergines and tomatoes, all containing solanine, may be an aggravating cause. Garlic is being increasingly recognized as a helpful food, both within the diet, and in tablet form. Some recommend cider vinegar, which is said to regulate the body's metabolism by entering the bloodstream, and dissolving the harmful acid deposits in body tissue. There are many diets recommended. None work for everyone; but everyone can find one that works for them. Obesity is known to make the problems worse.

Pain-killers should be avoided, as they can delay the cleansing effect of diet, as can stimulants such as coffee and tea, which contribute to the degenerative process, and reduce the absorbtion of calcium. Conversely, herbal teas, such as valerian, comfrey, camomile and parsley, are useful to arthritis sufferers. Smoking also aggravates the conditions.

For osteoporosis and osteomalacia, a diet containing calcium and protein from milk and calcium supplements is useful, but so is an efficient digestive system which ensures that the body absorbs calcium properly into the bones. If calcium is not so absorbed, it remains in the soft tissue where it can aggravate arthritic conditions, or hasten the hardening of arteries. Vitamin D from sunlight improves calcium assimilation, as does magnesium supplements. The tannin in tea can prevent the absorbtion of calcium.

Regular exercise is essential. First, research has shown that healthy animals, given adequate amounts of dietary calcium, continued to lose calcium from their bones if they were prevented from exercising. For calcium to be deposited in the bone, it has to be taken to it in the blood supply, a process increased by exercise. Second, exercise assists the normal functioning of joints, and avoids further deterioration by eliminating toxic wastes in the joints.

Alternative therapies

Alternative medicine offers different explanations, and different solutions for pain, which is essentially the outcome of toxicity. Older people, whose lives are racked with pain, should be advised to try other approaches. Alternative medicine may not deal with pain as quickly, for it realizes that the suppression of pain is a temporary expedient that can produce more serious long-term consequences, but there are many remedies and techniques which dampen pain, and do so with better long-term effectiveness, and fewer side-effects. Most alternative treatments attempt to reduce reliance upon pain-killers, but will do so sensitively, in recognition that people want to avoid pain wherever possible.

Most alternative practitioners recognize that arthritic pain is caused by faulty diet, and will recommend detoxifying diets which seeks to treat individual causation. Chronic pain sufferers can usefully consult with naturopaths, homeopaths, herbalists, acupunturists and osteopaths, all of whom have a positive record in the relief of pain.

Naturopaths recommend reducing the consumption of meat, including poultry, and increasing the consumption of fresh vegetables and fruit, with wholegrain cereals recommended for most individuals.

Homeopathic remedies seek to remove the toxicity that has built up in joints and muscles, with a wide selection of remedies which seek to identify and treat the individual's specific pain experience, principally rhus, tox, bryonia and ruta. Treatment will also address stress, diet, exercise and postural factors. Homeopathy is probably the best hope with osteoporosis, where treatment is usually effective, particularly if it is linked with the menopause.

Herbal remedies aim to support general vitality as well as deal with pain, focusing initially on exercise, nutrition and the elimination of waste products from the body. Herbalism can offer remedies such as devil's claw, which reduces inflammation, hawthorn which acts on the blood, and celery seed, which increases the elimination of acidity through the kidneys.

Many Oriental and manipulative therapies, particularly acupuncture, acupressure and reflexology, are noted for their effective pain relief. There are many reports indicating success in cases considered 'untreatable' by orthodox medicine. Acupuncture can reverse the degenerative changes of osteoarthritis, and is usually effective with rheumatism.

Exercise and postural therapies can be helpful in correcting postural faults, and relieving strain and tension. The Alexander principle deals with pain that has postural roots, and osteopathy has a proven record in acute cases. Yoga can also be beneficial, especially in remobilizing stiff and painful joints with its gentle, remedial exercises and positions, and in its ability to combat stress.

CANCER

Cancer is a malignant growth or tumour which distorts the process of cell division, leading to rapid proliferation, the invasion of neighbouring tissue and, ultimately, producing secondary growths throughout the body. Cancer can occur in the skin, glands, organs, muscles, bones and, as leukaemia, in the blood. It is an extreme example of the body's failure to maintain itself, as the immune system normally destroys cancerous cells, only failing when the body becomes weak, or troubled by strong emotional trauma or illness. For cancer to develop, there has to be a breakdown in normal health which allows cancer cells to multiply and spread, resulting in death when the level of tissue and organ destruction is no longer compatible with life.

Cancer is an increasing cause of death amongst all age-groups, and although older people are probably more susceptible to cancer, it tends to be less malignant, and grows more slowly than in younger people. Personality and lifestyle factors such as stress, smoking and diet, are causal factors, provoked by exposure to carcinogens, substances ranging from coal extract, asbestos fibre, lubricating oils, arsenic, some food additives and sweeteners. It is also caused by environmental factors, such as chemical pollution, radiation from ultraviolet light, X-rays, radioactivity used both in medicine and industry, and nuclear radiation from military sources and power generation.

Allopathic treatment

With the vast expenditure on cancer research, medicine is now claiming success in screening and identifying cancer. It is treated through chemotherapy, radiation and surgical removal. Chemotherapy utilizes highly toxic drugs, which are as dangerous to healthy tissue as to cancerous tissue. Radiation seeks to burn out the cancer, but can also destroy healthy surrounding tissue.

Some doctors have been highly critical of these methods. Richard (1982), a doctor involved in allopathic cancer treatment for 20 years, described the 'wanton suffering' caused by 'cut, burn and poison' techniques.

> Time and again a patient I'd known for years got cancer, was operated on and treated with radiation and drugs, and was returned to my care. The same routine then followed with remorseless repetition. I would begin the hopeless task of

presiding over that patient's decline, telling reassuring lies, and giving more and more pain-relieving drugs until death ensued. What about those who got better? There were not enough to write about.

Despite the increasingly sophisticated treatment, and growing medical claims, surgery, radiation and chemotherapy remain largely ineffective, perhaps even accelerating illness and death. There has to be considerable doubt whether such treatments represent the best long-term approach to tackling the problem of cancer. They do not play any role in its prevention and, with few exceptions, there is no convincing evidence that such treatment prolongs life, but abundant evidence that it reduces the quality of life.

The failure of treatment probably arises from its insistence that cancer is caused by 'rogue' cells, occurring by chance or misfortune, which can be treated by direct attack. Alternative therapies consider that cancer is the result of an unhealthy body experiencing an intolerable build-up of toxicity. Allopathy does not deal with this internal toxicity; indeed, radiation and chemotherapy are all drastic, highly toxic treatments that serve to further damage the immune system.

Prevention and alternative therapies

Alternative medicine believes that cancer is the consequence of careless lifestyle, and as such is a preventable disease. It is common for cancer sufferers to experience remission, during which time the cancer remains dormant. This can arise from the individual temporarily changing his or her lifestyle from the trauma of diagnosis, only for the disease to spread again when they return to previous practices.

There are general steps that individuals can take to prevent cancer, including the avoidance of known carcinogens, nicotine, tar, and alcohol, and the adoption of a healthy lifestyle. A sensible diet is usually recommended, free of excessive meat eating, preserved foods, caffeine (in tea, coffee and cola), and fried foods, but which includes large quantities of fresh food, including fresh fruits and vegetables, raw egg yolks, natural yoghurt, raw nuts and seeds. Passwater (1986) and Kidman (1983) describe in more detail the food hazards believed to contribute to the onset, and exacerbate the development, of different forms of cancer.

Mental attitudes are closely linked with cancer. Stress is a factor increasingly identified with cancer. The maintenance of a happy and fulfilling life, self-esteem and life-purpose, are important preventative factors, as is the ability to cope with anger, shock and grief. Another important precipitating factor in cancer is the loss of close friends and loved ones; but it is not loss, but the individual's response to loss, that is significant (Carlson, 1975).

Whilst no alternative therapy would claim definitive answers for treating cancer, most would argue that their methods were at least as effective, and certainly less discomfiting in their consequences than those conventionally applied. Alongside the increasing recognition of allopathic failure has arisen a corresponding interest in alternative approaches.

The main benefit of alternative therapies is to assist the body's immune system to defend itself effectively from cancer, both in preventing it occurring initially or, in re-establishing its natural power after cancer has been diagnosed. Both acupuncture and osteopathy can be used to treat pain often experienced in the back and shoulders, often associated with cancer of internal organs and, in doing so, is believed to improve the physiological functions which allowed it to develop initially.

There is considerable evidence that cancer follows severe emotional distress, indicating the power of the mind in the prevention and treatment of cancer. This is perhaps the basis for the success attributed to therapies based on relaxation, psychology and the paranormal. There are many techniques which have been found useful, including relaxation, mental imagery, meditation, hypnosis, including self-hypnosis, and autogenic training (Carlson, 1975).

Naturopathy is an important source of possible assistance, recommending strict dietary control and exercise, as both a preventative and remedial measure.

Homeopathy too offers a variety of remedies for the condition, which are said to be useful, particularly in the early stages of the disease.

Herbal remedies have a long and honourable history in the treatment of cancer (Hoffman, 1990), and although treatment focuses on the individual, there are a number of known antitumour herbs, some of which are now being properly researched, particularly in the USA.

MENTAL ILLNESS, DEPRESSION AND CONFUSION

Illnesses of the mind are the fastest growing health problem in the Western world. The neurological system controls all human activity.

Many illnesses arise directly from the mind, ranging from insomnia, loss of appetite, headache, migraine, neuralgia, tinnitus, vertigo, and other physical complaints; to depression and more serious psychiatric illness; and, ultimately, to memory impairment, confusion and dementia. Despite this, conventional medicine seeks to separate the mental from the physical, often suggesting that the mental is caused, or is remediable by, attention to physical factors.

Despite ageist misunderstandings, depression and mental decline are not age related. Everyone becomes depressed at times, this becoming a problem only when it becomes protracted, or when the reaction becomes disproportionate, in intensity or duration, to the situation being experienced. Most older people who suffer affective disorders are usually experiencing on-going mental health conditions experienced throughout life, although it is not uncommon for depression to result from the ageism that surrounds the ageing process.

Nor is severe memory loss and intellectual dysfunction an inevitable companion of ageing. Certainly, the ageing brain does deteriorate, yet whilst dementia usually affects older people, it also strikes younger people, some in their 40s, particularly those who consume a bad diet, or have suffered protracted mental stress. This gives a clue to the causes of dementia, but also indicates that the fundamental question should be why these physical changes occur, not when.

The impact of senility on older people is significant not just for those contracting the condition, but also those who fear the prospect of reduced mental capacity with ageing. The prospect of 'losing their mind' is perhaps the most powerful cause of the widespread fear of growing old. Most people would tolerate any physical loss rather than face life with a dysfunctioning mind. Our intellect is the custodian of our individuality. Once mental integrity is lost, we lose our human identity.

The pessimism of ageism, in which mental decline is an important element, can make dementia a self-fulfilling prophecy. Ageing is closely identified with feelings of being increasingly worthless, undervalued, lonely and depressed, not to mention the association with poverty and hardship. Yet most older people, and certainly those who do not accept the stereotypes of decline, can remain mentally active regardless of their age.

Indeed, severe depression can be mistaken for confusion, raising the interesting possibility that senility may result from the fear of senility.

Parkinson's disease This is a slowly progressive disease of the nervous system, characterized by shaking head and limbs, in which a movement requiring muscle control, such as eating, speaking and dressing, becomes progressively more difficult. It can eventually lead to constant stiffness, difficulty in walking, slurred speech, loss of memory, and considerable distress, anxiety and loss of confidence. Many older people will know the condition by its former name, 'the shaking palsy'. It is believed to be caused by the death of cells in the part of the brain which regulate voluntary movements, caused not by ageing, but by some kind of toxin or chemical. It has, for example, been linked with the use of herbicides in the environment, and is also known to result from the use of drugs, including the major tranquillizers.

Alzheimer's disease   The Alzheimer's brain has been found in post-mortem to have developed two abnormalities, neurofibrillar tangles, jumbled fibres found at nerve endings, and neuritic plaques, deteriorating pieces of nerve cells around a fibrous core. Both have been accepted as being at least the partial cause of the condition, although they have been found to be present in normal brains, leading to some scepticism about their significance (Monsour and Robb, 1982).

The disease is progressive, starting with forgetfulness, especially of short-term or recent memory, speech loss, and progressing to difficulty in undertaking simple tasks. This is followed by disorientation in time and place, and failure to recognize close friends. Ultimately, the personality changes, with formerly tranquil people becoming aggressive, even towards those caring for them; manners, social customs, and control over bodily functions are lost, with the individual losing interest in life, and eventually becoming totally dependent.

Arteriosclerotic dementia, or multiple infarct dementia   This condition is characterized by a stepwise deterioration of function, caused by a series of small strokes within the brain, themselves resulting from narrowed arteries in the brain, or clots, starving it of blood, and killing brain tissue. It can also be caused when blood vessels haemorrhage causing similar destruction of the brain.

There is progressive impairment of memory and logical thinking, loss of day-to-day household and intellectual skills; self-neglect, wandering, disorientation, inability to socialize, incontinence, difficulty in walking, feeding and dressing, and as brain damage is erratic, the course of illness fluctuates widely.

177

Allopathic treatment

Insomnia, anxiety, depression, schizophrenia and other mental conditions are treated with a variety of powerful drugs. Psychoactive drugs, such as sedatives, tranquillizers and antidepressants, embrace the main response to mental illness.

Tranquillizers are widely used. When they were introduced they seemed capable of changing moods, improving depression and paranoia, reducing unusual behaviour and the outward symptoms of distress, all with few side-effects. This led to their widespread prescription for a multitude of less serious emotional disturbances. They can effect emotional change, but there is no evidence that they are healing, and much that they can leave people withdrawn, apathetic and lacking in confidence. Long-term treatment, even in mild doses, can become addictive, and removing them can involve serious withdrawal symptoms.

Antidepressants are used to treat depression, anxiety, lack of sleep and agitation. Their side-effects are diarrhoea or constipation, dizziness, drowsinesss, fatigue, headache, vision disorders, heartbeat irregularities and low blood-pressure. Anticonvulsants are used for neuralgia, migraine and seizures. They can cause dizziness, drowsiness, nausea, blood disorders, lack of co-ordination, aggressiveness, insomnia, weakened bones, depression and fatigue. Antihistamines and antispasmodics are used in the treatment of nausea, vomiting, vertigo, anxiety, migraine, agitation and hearing disorders. They can cause confusion, drowsiness, blood disorders, dizziness and loss of appetite. Benzodiazepine and hypnotic drugs are used to treat nervous tension, anxiety, restlessness, insomnia and muscle spasm. They cause dizziness, drowsiness, fatigue, light-headedness, depression, digestive disorders, headache, and low blood-pressure, whilst with older people agitation and confusion are common.

The other drawback of psychoactive drugs is social rather than medical, in that they help people to tolerate intolerable situations, reducing their capacity to come to terms with, and challenge, what is happening in their lives. This is often based upon attitudes which suggest that older people should not feel emotional pain, should be protected from grief and, by doing so, removes from the individual an inviolable right to live and experience life as it is. Indeed, valium, librium and similar drugs have been prescribed for emotionally stable people suffering some temporary trauma, including many older people following bereavement. Such medication can interfere with the normal pattern of life, leading to further emotional disturbance, in an inability to come to terms with the reality of life, and possibly providing the basis for confusional states in later life.

Senility is often considered an unavoidable factor of ageing for which there is no cure. Certainly, there is no successful treatment for dementia. Parkinson's disease is treated by a number of drugs, notably levodopa, which do not cure the condition, or stop its progression. Their side-effects include constipation, diarrhoea, depression, anxiety, blood disorders, ulcers, heartbeat irregularity, nausea, dizziness, drowsiness and fatigue, and with prostate disorders and confusion being a particular problem for older people. Surgically, there has been some recent interest in the idea of brain cell implants. But, normally, people suffering dementia are left to sit out the rest of their lives.

The ageing brain is assaulted from many directions, not least the depression caused by ageing, and the toxic drugs that are prescribed to deal with their depression. There is now considerble evidence that confusion results from medication for other ailments, with many drugs known to cause confusional states. Older people tend to take more drugs, for more conditions, more regularly, than any other age group. Yet just as ageing people are more sensitive to drugs, the ageing brain is the most sensitive organ to drug reactions; it should not be surprising if it is the first system that breaks down when the drug burden becomes too great. The rapid rise in confusion is at least partially the result of increased toxic medication prescribed for older people.

Prevention

The links between mental health problems and old age are more closely associated with the social and emotional conditions in which older people live. Older people who have been cut off from mainstream social life, retaining no social role, few friends, few regular visitors, and little interest in the world about them, are particularly vulnerable. Structural ageism tends to diminish life opportunities, with the danger that older people are deprived of the mental stimulation necessary for maintaining a healthy brain. If older people do not retain stimulating intellectual interests, and maintain important social relationships, it makes them more susceptible to depression, which can lead to a crisis of identity, role and status, and to a deterioration in both physical and mental health. Ultimately, these factors may lead to the biochemical changes in the brain associated with dementia.

The maintenance of purpose and reason for living is a major objective in dealing with depression. Continuing intellectual demands should be made on older people. It is this that distinguishes people who remain mentally alert throughout old age. Whilst the ageing process will bring decline, the speed of that decline is, in many ways, under personal control. The key to successful ageing rests with the mental exercise provided by a rich and varied social environment. This has been demonstrated in laboratory experiments on rats, who were removed from solitary, uninteresting cages and placed in more challenging environments. Even older rats were able to form new brain connections, suggesting that brain cells can wither when life becomes dull and uninteresting, but that, regardless of age, they can grow and develop within a stimulating environment (Hunt, 1988). It was once thought that humans could not reproduce new nerve cells; but even this is now being challenged.

Good diet and adequate liquid consumption is vital, as even small nutritional deficiencies can have a major impact upon the brain and central nervous system, and many symptoms of malnutrition, including loss of appetite, fatigue, irritability, anxiety, depression, poor memory, insomnia, distractibility, and mild delusional states, resulting from dietary deficiency, can be mistaken for senility.

Psychodietetics has introduced the radical idea that many 'mental' and emotional problems are the result of improper nutrition, and that they can be prevented, treated and cured through nutrition. For example, an abnormal reduction in blood sugar level can affect the nervous system and brain, causing an erratic mental state with many symptoms, including dizziness, fainting, blackouts, headaches, fatigue, exhaustion, drowsiness, muscle pain, cramps, numbness, insomnia, nightmares, irritability, restlessness, nervous breakdown, lack of concentration, excessive worry and anxiety, depression, forgetfulness, illogical fears, suicidal thoughts, tremors, convulsions, neurodermatitis, loss of appetite, loss of sexual drive and impotency (Cheraskin et al., 1974).

Few people consider smoking a cause of emotional problems, yet nicotine, absorbed into the blood stream, adds to metabolic dysfunction by disturbing the digestive system, impairing vitamin C absorbtion, and interferes with blood circulation by constricting the blood vessels, thus robbing the brain of its supply of essential nutrients. In addition, caffeine, sugar, food additives and alcohol, can all cause problems either directly, or through impairing the body's ability to absorb the nutrients it requires.

Iatrogenic causes also have to be considered. Perhaps the first reaction to early signs of dementia should be to seek to eliminate, with the doctor's consent, all drugs for a trial period. This alone can sometimes alleviate the development of confusion, with an additional advantage being the discovery that an individual is able to manage on less drugs or, indeed, none at all.

Many other factors trigger depression, including dehydration, depression, environmental change, urine retention, constipation, pain and tumours of the lung. There is research which links Alzheimer's disease with brain damage caused by excessive alcohol consumption. It has also been suggested that aluminium, arising from its presence in food, dust and water, may play a part in the development of dementia. If so, excessive tea drinking must be another contributory factor, as Indian tea contains aluminium in significant quantities. Zinc deficiency, arising from inadequate diet, excessive alcohol, diuretic drugs, epilepsy and rheumatics drugs, have also been suggested as causative factors (Gidley and Shears 1988). Emotional stress, atmospheric pollution, and many other environmental factors, may also be important.

Any person who is not physically ill, but who manifests unusual emotional reactions, should look for the causes in four general areas (Watson, 1972):

1. inadequate nutrition;
2. chemical interference with the ability of tissues to function normally, owing to drugs, poisons, allergies or infections;
3. stress; and
4. failure to repair tissues because of lack of sufficient rest and sleep.

Alternative medicine

One advantage that alternative medicine has in treating mental and emotional disorders is that holistic therapies consider that an individual's state of mind and personal atittudes are an essential cause of illness, as well as a vital factor to be considered in treatment. Personality is considered the key to vitality, and resistance to illness. In this sense they are an important source of assistance.

However, no natural treatment has been found for dementia, except to recommend improvements in general health practices by attention to diet, exercise and reducing stress, particularly through naturopathy. It would be wrong to suggest that, at present, diseases of the brain are remediable through alternative medical means. Holistic medicine could perhaps provide a more important response, but the general neglect of demented older people extends to these disciplines as any other so, unfortunately, they remain a largely untested arena.

Homeopathy aims to relieve mental and emotional symptoms, and as remedies address personal emotions as well as physical illness, they are considered so important that they often point to the specific remedy to be used for most conditions. In this way, homeopathic treatments can assist people to change their responses to stress, anger and grief. For instance, when there is hardening of both body tissue and mental attitudes, nat mur and arsenicum can be helpful. For failing memory, Smith (1982) recommends lycopodium and baryta carb; and for mild confusional states, opium, baryta carb, cannabis, stramonium and belladonna. Those unable to relax can be helped by nux vomica, whilst ignatia is the remedy for problems of mourning and grief.

Herbalism is uniquely suited to treating the problems of nervous and emotional disorders, with Hoffman (1990) describing it as a 'co-operation between humanity, plants and the Earth in healing', with the action of herbs described in detail in Hoffman (1986). Vervain calms nervous irritability and exhaustion; passion flower and skullcap are relaxants, which induce more restful sleep; wild oats is a tonic that can calm the nervous system. One herb, ginkgo, is being studied for its value in Alzheimer's disease (Hoffman, 1990).

Aromatherapy can also recommend calming remedies, one being lavender; and acupuncture has been found to relieve trembling in Parkinson's disease. Mental conditions related to stress can benefit from medical therapies based upon relaxation, meditation and movement. Yoga is excellent, and Alexander technique, reflexology and other techniques using massage can also be helpful.

In conclusion, it is alway worth seeking advice about what self-help, prevention and alternative therapies can do with illness of all description. This has not been intended as a comprehensive list of ailments, but an indication of the value in broadening the horizons of medical responses to disease, its prevention, treatment and cure. There are a variety of other ailments, common with older people, that alternative medicine can usefully prescribe for, such as exhaustion, dizziness, insomnia, migraine, hay fever, palpitations, cramp, problems with eye-sight and hearing, indigestion, varicose veins, incontinence and psoriasis.

11

An approach to loss, death and dying

Loss is a lifetime experience. The earliest losses involve moving from our mother's body, followed by the incremental process of becoming a separate individual, the acceptance of the limits decreed by social convention, and the restrictions imposed by our personal abilities. As life progresses, there are losses concerned with our hopes, dreams and achievements, and our expectations of human relationships.

Loss in old age is often thought to constitute a problem of a different nature, quality and importance. Certainly, the experience of loss clusters significantly in later life, and bereavement and personal death are matters of immediate concern to older people, often profoundly. Yet they are not fundamentally different to those experienced throughout life. Loss can seem irreparable, leaving only sadness, pain and regret all with an inevitable certainty. Simone de Beauvoir (1966) traced the sorrows of old age from the first recorded lament through to the anguish of personal death, emphasizing the miseries of ageing. When ageing is seen in this way, it can appear to be the worst of misfortunes, worse even than death because it mutilates what we have been, whilst leaving us conscious of the damage.

Yet this ageist caricature of despair arising from loss does not necessarily reflect reality. It is not so much age, but individual personality and experience, that determines the response. Similar traumatic events can be variously interpreted by different individuals, never with indifference, but where consolation can remain, and the individual can continue to believe that the future is not entirely desolate. The problem which underlays loss is that mankind attempts to rationalize its own existence.

Man is gifted with reason; he is life being aware of itself . . .
This awareness of himself as a separate entity, the awareness of

his own short life span, of the fact that without his will he is born and against his will he dies, that he will die before those who he loves, or they before him, the awareness of his aloneness and separateness, of his helplessness before the forces of nature and of society, all this makes his separate, disunited existence an unbearable prison. He would become insane could he not liberate himself from this prison and reach out, unite ...

(Fromm, 1957)

There is a tendency to assume that death is the most important loss, yet for many older people it is not. Loss of work, income, financial security, status, role; the decline of manual and mental dexterity, sensory decline, the speed of reflexes, memory and concentration, can all impinge heavily on the lives of older people. There are particular losses for older women. Their experience is intensified by the identification of female beauty and sexual attractiveness with youth, ensuring that the older woman, living alone, is more vulnerable than the older man. Society is established so that most women lose their identity when their husbands die (Caine, 1975), with the social network of many bereaved women being compounded by poverty, as well as increasing physical insecurity.

However, it is the ultimate loss of death that will provide the main focus here, in the understanding that what can be learnt about dealing with death can be transferred to other losses. The loss of loved ones is known to be one of the most stressful, trauma-inducing events in life, but to varying degrees. Some older people respond to loss as an event that has to be accepted with regret, whilst others can become severely depressed, acting like helpless, hopeless and angry children. Many speak openly of death, and think endlessly about it. Others defy change, and resist all recognition that time is passing. Some desperately attempt to maintain their youth. Some envy young people their youth, eschewing the special qualities of old age. Others become bored and restless, others despairing or self-destructive. Some seek distraction in activity to the extent that they are unable to appreciate their own lives. Still others become depressed or embittered, denying the impending nature of death, persuading themselves that they alone might be able to cheat death. Others have suffered enough to welcome death, with some actively seeking it through suicide or euthanasia.

Where there is failure to cope with early losses, perhaps the loss of parents, the individual's ability to cope with future loss can be undermined. Loss in childhood tends to be suffered more sensitively than loss in later life. Certainly, older people with a previous record of poor mental or physical health tend to cope less satisfactorily with loss. Many other circumstances make loss particularly difficult to manage. Death through suicide is known to be especially onerous, and the mourning process is known to go awry when relationships have been either ambivalent or dependent. Perhaps more important, those who experience loss without support from close friends tend to suffer more intensely.

Regardless of the personal approach, it is the feeling of inevitability and personal devastation caused by loss that needs to be avoided. There is no evidence that older people should be more worried by grieving. Many people do not actually fear death so much as the way they might effect the life-death transition. Indeed, the experience of ageing can enhance the development of new strengths, such as wisdom, candour and honesty, a wider perspective, and greater toughness, which can all assist in dealing with loss.

Yet even if older people remain confident and healthy, they must tackle the dominant social attitudes which consider them to be sexless, useless, powerless and a social burden. Ageism is designed to fulfil itself, fashioning ageing as a time of unremitting decline, during which occupation and vigour is lost, and friends become seriously ill and die. Older people, particularly those suffering from chronic illness, are perceived to be a burden for which death is often seen as the solution of an uncomfortable social problem. These perceptions have defined the way that ageing, bereavement and death are viewed, contributing to the idea that loss becomes inevitable, unpalatable and totally traumatic. Then death ceases to be an event to be tackled at an individual, human level, but something to be avoided.

Loss in old age, particularly through the death of loved ones, can be a major cause of stress, which in turn can have a harmful effect on mental and physical health. Worry increases pain, and can initiate illness. Many survivors of major loss contract disease, have accidents, become severely depressed, resort to smoking and drinking, quickly die or commit suicide, all at a higher rate than otherwise.

Yet this does not have to be so. Loss is not a unitary experience, nor is it an illness, or a painful precursor of death. Nor should it necessarily increase susceptibility to illness. The value of good friends, an optimistic personality, and an adequate income are factors which certainly make loss easier to accept. Ultimately, it is personal attitudes as much as the nature of loss which will determine the quality of recovery. Those who survive best are those with a healthier attitude to loss; how this can be achieved is an important aspect of healthy ageing.

The first prerequisite of a healthy approach to death and dying is to provide older people with the information to make an informed choice. It should not be a simple question either of hoping for immortality, or becoming resigned to fate. The third, more acceptable choice, involves a realistic openness, honesty, and acceptance of death, not an acceptance which removes the need for personal resolve, but one which recognizes that preparations have to be made.

Episodes of loss constitute periods of transition, of which death is the final one. Throughout life, individuals endeavour to lay down structures for their life by making key choices and pursuing specific goals. Many find it difficult to accept that their life, and all they have striven to create and enjoy, will finish. Yet it is so; even when the individual believes that some element of self will survive into eternity, life as we know and experience it remains transient, and will eventually be obliterated.

Even the most optimistic people have to acknowledge that ageing does involve losses which have to be accepted. Any transition from one stage to another implies an ending, a process of separation from what was previously important. Each should lead to an examination of how the new stage is to be tackled, requiring an examination of the nature of the losses involved which raise realistic questions about them, and an exploration of future prospects.

Accepting the inevitability of death requires that it is placed within a framework which gives it meaning and significance, not easy within contemporary culture. Prevailing attitudes towards loss in old age, particularly towards death, are unhealthy and mistaken. Death has become a taboo subject. Aries (1983) said that our culture tries to deny the very existence of death, writing dramatically of 'death being driven into secrecy'. Kubler-Ross (1973) argued that death has become a 'dreaded and unspeakable issue in our society'. Sontag (1983) found that lying to cancer patients 'is a measure of how much harder it has become in advanced societies to come to terms with death'. The outcome is often to undermine the honesty of final communication between friends, transforming grief from an endurable time of regret and sadness, to an agonizing nightmare.

Dominant social ideas, particularly religious and medical ideas, have led to uncertainty about coping with loss. Either a fatalistic attitude develops, with the ageist acquiescence to fate that this implies, or the raising of fanciful ideas of immortality, or significantly increased longevity. The inadequacy and decline of religious beliefs, and the failure of religious ceremonies to offer real help, has not been matched by the development of secular replacements. Some writers,

(Bohm, 1981; Capra, 1975; Lovelock, 1979; Sheldrake, 1987) have explored interpretations in which many levels of meaning attach to commonplace events. Dying becomes a transition from one level of meaning and existence to another, seeking to dignify dying when that becomes inevitable, and give it a positive purpose. The aim is to allow the individual freedom to relinquish life gracefully, instead of clinging to life at all costs. Time should not be measured as the period left to live, but to accept the next stage of life as a time of potential, and look positively at what it might offer. Ultimately, it means that close friends can live fully right up to the point of death, and where the wake becomes a celebration, without funereal misery.

This is not the normal approach, which has seen the development of many psychological mechanisms which determine the way individuals face bereavement. Foremost amongst these is denial, which has significant implications for older people, who are increasingly aware of their own mortality; To deny death is to disavow an important part of the ageing experience, both for the bereaved, and those who seek support and comfort in their own terminal decline. It restricts the expression of important emotions that are a necessary part of coming to terms with events; weeping has become synonymous with hysteria, and mourning with being morbid. Too much emotion is something to be avoided, with damaging results.

> They have no-one to talk to about the only subject that matters
> to them, the person they have lost. There is nothing left for
> them to do but die themselves, and that is often what they do,
> without necessarily committing suicide.
>
> (Aries, 1983)

The act of dying is now probably a lonelier event than ever before. Mourning and funerals are more discreet and muted than formerly. Aries (1983) affirms that dying was once experienced not only in association with friends and relations, but with other members of the community. Now Aries believes that we have 'removed death from society, eliminated its character of public ceremony, and made it a private act'. Described elsewhere is the technical perfection that has been achieved in transferring the corpse from the death bed to the grave, a process by which the dying are discretely removed from social life.

Younger people, including professional carers, dismiss remarks made by older people indicating that they are thinking about death. Discussing loss and death is avoided because it is believed to be a painful subject. Such thoughts are usually considered to be a painful subject. Such thoughts are usually considered to be unnecessarily morbid, although the truth is often that they are probably more painful for younger people than those who more imminently and personally face the prospect of decline and death. It is thought safer to abstain from thoughts of death, proceeding with life by refusing to deal with the anxieties and grief that loss engenders. For older people, the taboo can lead to many difficulties, including an inability to prepare for, and to come to terms with, the realities of ageing, physical and mental decline, and ultimately with death itself.

Older people also practise denial, forgetting that no one can retain their youth, that time cannot be stopped, and that human relationships do not last forever. Denial might make it appear easier to live oblivious to the realities of loss, but as Freud and later psychologists have argued, denial can eventually impoverish the experience of life. Too much psychological energy is consumed deflecting fears of death, and replacing them with other anxieties. Ongoing denial, and the unresolved emotions of anxiety, sadness and despair is not only painful, but can have a devastating effect on the psychological and physical health of older people.

> Give sorrow words; the grief that does not speak
> Whispers the oe'r fraught heart, and bids it break.
>
> (Shakespeare, *Macbeth*, Act 4, scene 3)

The outcome of denial, both for the dying and the bereaved, is that death often arrives suddenly, a trauma for which people are unprepared. This is both unnecessary and unfortunate. Whilst we may be powerless to prevent loss, we can develop strategies that can protect from the pain of separation. Yet even though it is neither sensible or possible to stop time, denial is endemic. In order to deal with it, it is helpful to look at the ideas that form the foundation of the denial of death in modern society.

Religious ideas

Religious teaching informs us that death is not final. The religious legacy of Christianity includes the familiar images of resurrection, immortality, the imperishable soul, life after death, and the promise that death will lead to eternal, blissful reunion with those we love. Whilst these do not necessarily deny our mortal death, they do indicate that death is not final.

> I am the resurrection and the life, says the Lord. If anyone believes in me, even though he dies, he will live. Anyone who lives and believes in me, will not die, alleluia.
>
> (John 11:25–6)

Implicit in all religious teaching, especially Christian and Islamic teaching, is a tendency to devalue the significance of dying. Where there is life after death, the importance of death is discounted.

This feeds ageism by leading younger people to dismiss, and older people to accept, death as a natural process, one that should be faced with joy and expectation. It discounts the personal issues involved with this world, indicating that feelings about loss and death should be considered of central importance. Religion has replaced clear thinking about the nature of death with ideas concerning rebirth in some other form. This can be reincarnation, or living on through nature, the oceans, mountains, trees, or ascending into Heaven. All serve as images of immortality. We die, but the Earth, or Heaven continues, allowing us to live through history, through our genes, our children and descendants.

The widespread assumption that religion is a source of solace for the bereaved and the dying should be questioned. Freud argued that 'the consolation of the religious illusion' was unhelpful, believing that religious dogma is based upon illusions built up by many to make the helplessness of the individual in this world incurable. He felt that just as children depend on their parents to protect them, so anxious adults depend on gods, that we create religion to 'exorcise the terrors' of nature, to make up for the sufferings that civilization imposes, and to reconcile ourselves to the cruelty of our fate, particularly as it is shown in death.

All religions have a vested interest in death, but their function is to sanctify it, and to give meaning to what has occurred by reference to what is to come in the hereafter. Contrary to popular perception, religion does not help people come to terms with the social and emotional realities of the present, and does not pretend to do so.

Medical ideas

Medicine is introducing an extension to the religious denial of death. Surgery already replaces hearts, lungs, kidneys and other bodily parts. We are led to believe that medical science will ultimately vanquish illness; even if, unintentionally, medicine raises expectations of 'miracle cures', eventually perhaps for death itself, not just in a supernatural, but a mortal sense.

Death is seen as unacceptable, not a 'natural' event, but one that will eventually be cured. In the USA, one-third of medical expenditure is directed towards people with less than a year to live (Gidley and Shears, 1988). It is not ageist to argue that this should not happen, for keeping a dying individual alive at all costs, particularly someone who might prefer to die, is a denial of dignity and humanity, and an obstruction to the process of coming to terms with decline and death. Many dying people in the USA have their bodies frozen by cryonics companies in the hope that medical science might eventually be able to cure their condition so that they can be thawed, and brought back to life. Other people have been persuaded that lavish doses of nutrients can extend life, perhaps to eternity. It is possible that some people who strive for physical immortality are motivated by a love of life and a faith in science; but most are driven by the terror and denial of death.

The medical quest for immortality, the belief that science will eventually conquer problems relating to illness, have other consequences. Given these unrealistic expectations, death can be seen as a medical failure, making it profoundly disturbing for doctors who are repeatedly confronted with it. This challenges medicine either to review the effectiveness of dominant attitudes and technology, which is often refused, or to discount or marginalize death. Faced with this choice, ageing provides a useful alibi for failure, and an interesting dichotomy develops in which the implicit medical promise of immortality faces the medical neglect of ageing, and the discounting of illness in old age. Both ideas are damaging to the interests of older people: the first promises the unattainable, the second leads to ageist neglect. Combined, they lead to the kind of modern, technological medical care of older people often witnessed.

The medical struggle to avoid death often leads to life being prolonged to the detriment of individual dignity and comfort (Parkes, 1972). Yet the denial of death can simultaneously lead to the emotional support for the dying patient being neglected. Intensive medical care is often insensitive to the needs of terminally ill people, and their close friends. The distinction between the importance attached to the physical care of dying people, in the form of treatment that prevents death but does not enhance life, and the emotional care given to older people is often conspicuous. Hospital routine concentrates on bodily care to the detriment of emotional needs, particularly during the final stages of dying. Equally, for the bereaved, there is a marked tendency 'to prescribe pills rather than give supportive care to the bereaved' (Bowling and Cartwright, 1982).

Our lack of preparation for death is part of a wider problem in which death is rarely perceived as a natural event, but is invariably experienced 'as an unjustifiable violation' (de Beauvoir, 1966). Yet postponing death at any age creates ethical problems (Dubos, 1970). To save children is considered a humane act; but its consequence is often to intensify future medical requirements. Prolonging the life of sick older people has to be measured against the quality of future life expectations, and the hardships that medicalized survival entails for the individual, the family, and the costs borne by the community. The postponing of death from irreversible illness necessitates the provision of exacting medical supervision essentially in an attempt to avoid the unavoidable. By sanctifying physical life through the evasion of death, rather than by maintaining health and, ultimately, accepting death when it becomes unavoidable, we create expectations that are impossible to deliver.

What is required is not a cure for death, but an improved attitude towards it. Living and dying are partly dependent upon the will to live, which can be assessed by asking people to rate their keenness to carry on living, and Argyle (1987) found that the will to live is much reduced in those who are socially isolated, in poor health, or who feel that they have lost their usefulness. Awareness of mortality, both ours and other people's, can heighten appreciation of life without necessarily making death acceptable.

Yet openness in bereavement and death has also been criticized. The concept of 'apologism' has been described by Walford (1983), who believes that it is possible to achieve a significant extension of human lifespan. He argues that resistance to increased longevity is rooted in attitudes that make it impossible either because it is against the Divine Order, or which insists that the destiny of all animals is to die. Apologism is identified with ideas that believe that there can be no birth without death, that procreation must preclude immortality, that the Earth could not sustain both reproduction and eternally living beings, that death is important in order to make room for new generations. It would also lead to social stagnation, and the natural process of evolution, in which death is necessary for the development of any species, would be harmed. This is why all creatures have a maximum lifespan, genetically programmed to die. Apologism believes that science should not meddle in life, and hence with death. Immortality is undesirable as people would become devastatingly wrinkled, decrepit, and senile, or just overwhelmingly bored.

Writers who have challenged the taboos, lies and deceptions surrounding death have been branded as 'apologists'. In Walford's terms, Kubler-Ross (1973) is an apologist whose belief that dying can be a beautiful experience, and that dying is the last big growth experience of human life, is interpreted as being against the move to increased human longevity.

This confuses two issues. Walford believes that life can be extended, and is critical of ideas that lead to individuals becoming resigned to death. Yet he does not deny that death will occur, and should not deny that people need to be prepared for it. The two ideas are not mutually exclusive. It is unnecessary to become resigned to death on the basis of chronological age alone. It is possible to extend the length and quality of life far longer into old age than is currently achieved. Yet the acceptance of death is unnecessary, whether at 70 or 80 as conventionally believed, or at 120, as Walford believes is possible.

Timing is the essence of the difficulty. The will to live, and a sensible strategy for extending health, does not preclude an acceptance of decline and death. Indeed, accepting the entire process of life, including death, is an essential part of healthy living.

THE MOURNING PROCESS

Mourning is the process by which individuals adapt to the losses of life, acknowledge the pain it produces, feel it, and live past it. Freud said that mourning consists of a slow, difficult, extremely painful process of letting go. Mourning is usually about death of people we love; but we need to mourn many social and physical losses, such as the end of a marriage, or special friendships. The deeper, more meaningful the nature of the loss, the deeper the mourning.

The ability to mourn is essential for older people who have a declining number of people to love. Yet whilst there are many losses in old age, another, more hopeful view is that if we mourn the losses of ageing properly, it can lead to further development, and an ability to embrace life.

Mourning has to be more than an exercise, acknowledged by the intellect but denied with the emotions. Intellectualizing often takes the form of reciting religious phrases, fantasizing about the past, searching for the dead, and trying to deny the finality of loss, all of which does little to remedy the losses entailed. It is the emotional and social losses that are the most devastating. Viorst (1986) asserts that the death of a spouse involves losing an entire social unit, including a companion, lover, intimate friend, protector and provider, all requiring replacement. The appalling loneliness that results can make the future seem worthless.

One problem with mourning is a tendency to idealize the dead, suspending criticism, with past misdeeds overlooked. The funeral oration talks of nothing which is unfavourable.

Consideration for the dead, when it is no longer required, is often greater than it was during their lifetime. One unintended consequence is for survivors to feel that their prospects for the future are even less tolerable.

For these and other reasons, the process of mourning can go awry. When faced with bereavement, there is a danger that the individual remains stuck in the mourning process. It is difficult to provide time-limits for mourning; but in time it is important that the individual is willing to let go of the lost relationship. Mourning becomes pathological when it is doggedly retained, when holding on to grief feels like fealty, and giving it up like betrayal of the dead. In prolonged or chronic mourning, individuals become paralysed in a state of intense, unremitting grief, clinging without relief to sorrows, anger, guilt, self-hatred or depression, unable to proceed with the rest of life.

Kubler-Ross (1973) urged a more open dialogue with those who are terminally ill, outlining an approach to counselling bereaved and dying people which sought to take them through five stages of grief, namely, denial, anger, bargaining, depression and acceptance. After this, mourning ceases, although there will still be regret, times when the dead are missed; this will accompany a gradual process of recovery, acceptance and adaptation.

Every individual, regardless of age, is capable of recovering stability, hopefulness, a capacity to enjoy life, and an acceptance that the dead will not return. Indeed, it is when the present and future continue to have value that the experience of ageing is enhanced. Loss should never be dwelt upon; instead, ageing people should learn to utilize fully the time available to them. The main choice survivors have concerns what to do with the dead: to die when they die; to live on impaired; or to fashion from the pain and memory a new life. Through mourning we let the dead go, and come to accept the difficult changes that loss brings.

Medicine can obstruct the grieving process. The introduction of 'new' illnesses, for example, 'delayed traumatic shock', serves only to medicalize the process of mourning, and explain why people fail to emerge successfully from it. 'Illness' is used to explain and justify holding on to feelings of grief and injustice; it is no longer necessary for the individual to emerge from grief bcause medicine has diagnosed the condition as an illness. Our feelings become medicalized; we no longer have to accept responsibility, which passes to medical professionals.

Older people can live a fuller and healthier old age, if they accept the inevitability of death, whilst at the same time maintaining a determination to delay 'old age' by adopting healthy lifestyles. How the older individual deals with loss is a vital component of this. But growing old, and dealing with loss, can be accomplished more gracefully if social involvement is maintained. Everyone needs contact with people, interests and enterprises as an insurance against becoming bored, or boring, or both. Living is a continuous process of feeling, loving and letting go. This struggle should never cease, for it helps the older individual adjust to losses which would otherwise appear irreplaceable. It is important that people consider and discuss personal attitudes to important matters, particularly those which they face with trepidation and fear, regularly revising them as experience requires.

It is also important to remember that pleasure does not lose its value in old age. Indeed, with less responsibility, old age can be a time when complete hedonism becomes possible. However, with increasing loss, many older people may find that they require more than this, in particular, a capacity for what is called ego transcendence.

Ego transcendence recognizes that life is finite, but allows us to make connections with the future through people and ideas which pass beyond personal mortality by means of some legacy that can be left to the next generation. It involves a capacity to delight in the pleasures of other people, a capacity to concern ourselves with events not directly related to personal self-interest, but a capacity to invest in tomorrow's world that we will not know. As grandparents, teachers, social reformers, collectors or creators of art, we can endeavour to leave an intellectual, spiritual, material or physical legacy which can constructively deal with the grief felt over the ultimate loss of self.

Looking back over life can also be helpful. Reminiscence can help the individual recall the important times and experiences of personal history. The life review is a summing up, a final integration between the past, present and future. Examining the part we are engaged in is the central task of Erikson's eighth and final age, ego transcendence. If this is to lead to 'integrity' rather than disgust and despair, individuals have to accept that we have a single life cycle, and that we must seek to find meaning and value in it. We have to accept 'the fact that one's life is one's own responsibility' (Erikson, 1971).

OUR OWN LOSSES, AND DEATH

Everyone will eventually need to mourn their own personal death. This is the final transition. Throughout our lifetime, the way we perceive others, and the physical changes within ourselves, will confirm that earlier definitions of 'self' have needed to be redefined.

Each stage ensures that we relinquish former images, replace them with others, and move on. Finally, we have to learn that no matter what we do to maintain health, we will eventually die. There is no immortality.

How should we relinquish our mortality? The concept of the 'good death' has been redefined drastically in recent times. Instead of being a conscious and expected end, as it was throughout ancient times, it is now considered to be what used to be a shameful death; sudden, striking without warning, and happening quietly in sleep. Generally, people face death in accordance with their personality, dying as they have lived. Those with spirit die with spirit. Those who lived impassively die impassively. Those who have denied reality continue to deny the imminence of death. Those who have always feared loss will die in terror.

It is increasingly common for people to die surrounded by denial. Glaser and Strauss (1965) referred to four circumstances in which death occurs:

1. Closed awareness is a situation in which individuals fail to recognize impending death, even though everyone else does.
2. Suspected awareness happens when the individual suspects what other people know, and attempts to confirm or invalidate the suspicion.
3. Mutual pretence awareness occurs when each party knows that death is imminent, but each pretends to the other that it is not so.
4. Open awareness is a situation where everyone is aware of approaching death, and acts honestly upon this awareness.

There is no easy answer to the problem. Some people believe that unspoken, private fears of death are worse than shared and certain knowledge that it is so. Yet there are many barriers of fear erected between doctors, dying people and relatives. In some cases, people dying with cancer are told they have 'ulcers', or some non-terminal ailment. It is hard to translate a theoretical 'right to information' into practice, sensitively interpreting what the individual wants to know. Often, uncertainty on the part of carers about what to say places the sick person in a difficult and cruel situation.

New approaches to the psychology of dying are being developed with the terminally ill, both in hospices and amongst those who have chosen to spend their last days with their families and friends. Counsellors working in this field have discovered that patients are able to come to terms with the situation once the initial fear has been eliminated (Hope, 1989). The hospice movement attempts to provide compassionate care allied with pain relief for dying people, without any pretence that there is a possibility of extending life. This model of care does not regard death as a 'failure' of medicine, but a natural process which requires sensitive care. It is based on the idea that honesty is vital, allowing the individual to ask questions, and discuss his or her fears openly. The disease takes second place to the social and emotional needs of the individual, in contrast to the slow, lonely process of dying in a hospital bed, plugged into tubes and machines which seek to maintain physical life. The family is also encouraged to become part of the process, and they, too, are helped to prepare for bereavement prior to death, redefining the 'good death' as one where there is time to experience dying.

There is always a need to make positive preparations for dying, making known personal wishes about funeral arrangements, and planning for those who will be left behind.

There are also problems associated with personal wishes concerning death. Attempted suicide amongst older people is less common than in younger people, although completed suicide rates increase with age, especially with men. Euthanasia remains an emotive subject guaranteed to raise many ethical questions. Both raise questions about whether the problems of old age, and personal death, should be met with acceptance and resignation, or should be resisted and fought, and when one should begin and the other end.

What needs to be realized, particularly by those who condemn both, is that old age can undoubtedly become dominated by suffering, and made unendurable by loss. Life can become a ceaseless struggle in a world which no longer offers sufficient reason to continue living.

One view of suicide and euthanasia is that it is a revolt against death, a healthy approach involving an acceptance of death without bitterness. Certainly, many older people do not consider death to be an enemy, but a friend. It offers the chance to relinquish their burden, whether that burden is caused by grief arising from loss, the pain of degenerative disease, the torment of terminal illness, or the feelings of helplessness, uselessness, and loneliness in old age.

12

The role of the professional carer

AGEING, HEALTHY AND IN CONTROL

Carers can play a significant role in the health of older people. Many questions have been raised concerning dominant attitudes towards health in old age and, in particular, the role of orthodox medical practice. The primary role of the carer arising from this assessment is to enable the individual to reassume personal control over his or her health, redressing the power balance between the individual and medical professionals, always emphasizing the non-medical aspects of health care, and encouraging prevention and self-care.

Professional intervention falls short of providing this role for older people, not least because the potential for doing so has not been seriously considered. Indeed, social workers and others have continued to express ambivalence towards working with older people.

> Professional social workers, like others, found it hard to accept the limited goals, inevitable deterioration, and the need for continuing service in work with old people.
>
> (Younghusband, 1978)

A range of studies (summarized in Goldberg and Connelly (1982)) have criticized two particular aspects of social work which narrow the focus of intervention. First, there has been a failure to identify signs of social and psychological distress. Second has been the low priority accorded to work with older people.

Ageism, particularly, presents major obstacles to the development of more positive and imaginative work. Social workers, like other professional groups, hold essentially negative attitudes about working with older people.

Social workers are not alone. Health visitors have a preventive focus with both children and older people, but their work with the latter is considered a low priority. The role of district nurses in family care should consist of both nursing and educational elements, but the educational role has been obscured by nursing demands to the extent that district nurses have developed an even more practical approach than health visitors, and their preventive work with older people is minimal. The increase in wardened, or sheltered housing, accommodation has also presented opportunities, but the role of wardens remains contentious between those who take a helping, but non-intrusive 'good neighbour' approach, and those who advocate a more proactive, preventative role. Most wardens have become pre-occupied with the day-to-day illnesses and crises, missing the opportunity for developing interventions which would provide tenants with a sense of empowerment (Phillipson and Strang, 1984).

The result is that medical staff undertake little preventive work with older people. They face the constraint of working within the conventional medical establishment, which is unlikely to welcome a wider approach to health which undermines its own central role. Yet this problem should not be insuperable. More significant are professional attitudes which believe there is limited scope for tackling issues connected with an ageing population.

These attitudes are manifest in professional training, arising from pressures within an over-crowded curriculum, and negative attitudes on the part of both staff and students. Large areas of neglect at all levels of social work training have been found, including nutrition, physical fitness, home safety, the prevention of hypothermia, sexuality, and the health needs of ethnic minority elders. (Phillipson and Strang, 1986).

Yet if professional carers fail to address the problems of ageism, family carers are even less likely to do so, as professional attitudes are influential in shaping and perpetuating images and beliefs about the ageing process amongst the general population. The major role of caring for older people is undertaken by thousands of unpaid relatives and friends, and the impact their attitudes have towards the task of looking after older people is crucial. Many older people, and their carers, have low expectations about health in old age, and these feelings are too often reinforced in encounters with professional staff.

Professionalisation has stifled the development of a perception that physical and mental aspects of ageing can be controlled both by judicious use of the health and welfare system and strategies for self-health care and self-help care.

(Phillipson and Strang, 1984)

The result is a lack of imaginative work with older people, with workers becoming depressed by the prospect of routine visits for assessment and surveillance, whilst witnessing what appears to be inevitable decline. Such innovation may be prevented by organizational difficulties, but more is concerned with deeply ingrained ageist attitudes. Older people remain ageing, unhealthy and not in control.

TACKLING AGEISM

Changing professional attitudes could have an important impact upon the approach to the task, and the morale of those undertaking it. Caring for older people within an ageist context is bound to be problematical, but to rise above ageist constraints requires more than good intentions. Sympathy is a necessary prerequisite for empathy, but taking a benign interest in older people can involve a subtle mixture of diminution and patronage, and the risks of 'welfarising' them (Bhadura, 1989). This arises when carers do not allow older people their full human stature, who become instead the objects of pity to be patronized.

Publicly funded social services are more than systems for distributing services; they are systems of social relationships that select and bolster power inequalities between experts and lay persons, as well as being providers and recipients of service ... Service strategies in general, and those for the aged in particular, tend to stigmatize their clients as recipients in need, creating the impression that they have somehow failed to assume responsibility for their lives. The needs of older persons are reconceptualized as deficiencies by the professionals charged with treating them, regardless of whether the origins of these needs lie in social conditions over which the individual has little or no control, in the failings of the individual, or in some policy-maker's decision that a need exists.

(Estes, 1979)

The myth of philanthropy indicates that harmful consequences can flow from good intentions. The rapid growth of professional care has arisen without any deep appreciation of the needs of older people. It has been characteristic by professional assumptions that were believed to be in touch with the emotional and material needs of their clients, and that possessed adequate 'theoretical' knowledge about the social and biological construction of old age (Phillipson and Strang, 1986).

A tougher approach, more sensitive to the real needs of older people, more capable of distinguishing between ageing and ageism is required. A willingness to confront ageist practice is essential, and must arise from antiageism training, and the development of an antiageist approach to illness which seeks to unravel the psychology that assumes that illness and old age are inevitable companions. Moreover, it is an approach which has to be achieved with both older people, and their carers.

For carers to escape from stultifying ageist assumptions, it is vital that they question their personal motivation, and examine their own ageism. Ageist attitudes constitutes a major disincentive to the development of radical practice. Too many professional staff are stuck in an approach which emphasizes the least attractive, malfunctioning features of ageing. This invariably focuses upon old age as a social problem, linking it with perspectives of the growing demographic burden, and loose notions of a 'rising tide of mental and physical frailty' (Phillipson and Strang, 1986). Dependency and disability are foremost – these usually assumed to be the result of biological ageing rather than socially constructed phenomena.

In working with older people, it is necessary to do more than meet immediate needs, instead concentrating on the importance of raising consciousness about ageist social assumptions.

> Consciousness raising goes beyond the promotion of positive images to the critical evaluation of the sources of negative images in societal dynamics. Like the women's movement, the old people's movement might question and analyze, and thereby begin to defuse, cultural messages about old age and the pervasive emphasis on youth and physical appearance.
>
> (Furstenberg, 1989)

DEMEDICALIZING OLD AGE

Life in old age can remain a fulfilling and rewarding experience, without significant loss of either physical or mental capacity. People in advanced old age can remain relatively free from illness; indeed, the majority of older people retain a reasonable standard of health.

This suggests that when older people do suffer from 'elderly ailments', their condition should be considered abnormal, just as it should do for any other generation.

Caring staff with responsibility for older people should begin to take a more active role, particularly within the powerful and influential medical profession. The first step is simply to challenge the doctors, many of whom would already agree that they do not have all the answers, and that they probably do as much harm as good. Such challenges alter the skewed power structure that exists within the growing partnership between the health and social services, a partnership which may well be encouraged by the new GP contracts, with their increased emphasis on preventive measures.

This does not necessarily initiate confrontation with the medical profession, even though it disqualifies the idea that 'the doctor knows best'. A wider approach can become a positive partnership involving a network of people, all contributing their particular insight and skill, eventually leading to a reduction in medication.

To date, there has been a lack of confidence in asking such questions, let alone attempting to play a more active role. Social workers, in particular, have remained content to be a junior partner to the medical establishment. Social work, when it adopts an holistic approach, offers the potential to be centrally involved in health care. There are many examples of non-medicalized approaches to health, but two examples might suffice to demonstrate its potential.

The health education project, undertaken by Pensioners Link in Barnet, was based on a wider understanding of elderly health. Its courses consisted of a series of talks and activities for older people, designed to improve their knowledge, understanding and awareness of health matters, and aimed to encourage them to take preventative measures in their own health care. The project found that such courses had a significant impact on older people, particularly when they became active participants. The main conclusion was that preventative work should be recognized as a priority, and that traditional patterns of health education for older people should be challenged (Meade, 1986).

The 'well-woman' approach is now being developed by groups of older people. First, there is the attempt to define ageing as a normal event, and to challenge its presentation as an illness and deviation from a well-established path. Secondly, there is an attempt to restore to older people knowledge and control of the ageing process. The parallels with the women's movement are clear. Older people must be recognized to have skills and abilities which can be utilized to ensure that growing old is a positive and affirmative experience. Depriving older people of the necessary health and social care skills makes positive ageing much harder to achieve (Phillipson and Strang, 1986).

The need to recognize iatrogenesis is not just a medical task. Indeed, it cannot be left to any single group. Those who spend most time with an individual are in the best position to recognize it. In descending order of importance, the individual is clearly most important, with daily carers second, and regular visitors third. Doctors come way down the list, prescriptions usually being made swiftly, on a monthly or longer basis, particularly with repeat prescriptions.

The relationship between social and medical factors in old age will become increasingly important, but it has to be a relationship based on equality, not one of 'master-servant'. It will involve recognizing iatrogenesis, questioning the need and effectiveness of medical treatment, and reducing the medication prescribed to older people wherever possible. The boundaries between what belongs to the individual, what belongs to the medical practitioners, and the potential role of carers, needs to be seriously rethought.

AN HOLISTIC APPROACH

Professional carers should be able to take a wider, structural view of the health of older people. Seeing older people in terms of their immediate problems and needs presents a pathological model of ageing which fails to acknowledge the wider picture, as the view is inevitably dominated by illness, disability, deprivation, decline and death.

When older people become ill, it should be possible to look beyond illness as a 'mechanical' problem, best treated with drugs and other palliatives. Old people are complex individuals and many facets have to be considered. The underlying cause of illness should be sought, based on an understanding of the total life of the individual, and a remedy found from knowledge available in many quarters.

When social and environmental factors are considered, the maintenance of health becomes something in which every individual has a role, but none more centrally than carers. The wider definition of good health defined by the World Health Organization, as 'a positive state of physical, mental and social well-being, not merely the absence of disease and infirmity' indicates that health is associated with many more factors than medical practitioners would normally consider, and moves attention from medication to the provision of social, emotional and environmental care.

The idea of caring for older people within the totality of their lives is attractive. A wider appreciation of the causation of illness, which assimilates the role that poverty, bereavement, social isolation, loneliness, status and role, loss, handicap, apathy and abuse, play in the lives of older people is particularly suited to social work philosophy.

> The social worker is ... concerned with remedying certain deficiencies which may exist in the relation between the individual and his environment, and for this purpose is concerned with the total individual in relation to the whole of the environment, in so far as this is relevant to righting such deficiencies.
>
> (Younghusband, 1951)

Social work is not restricted to one specific aspect of life, as is medicine and health, or education and the intellect. It is able to observe the individual functioning within their total environment. A more recent assessment of the potential role of the social worker, raising the possibility of understanding the problems and circumstances of people's life holistically has been presented by Jones (1983).

> Social work allows for perspectives that are not simply shaped and determined by economistic and commercial considerations, and that include a consideration of human needs, emotions and feelings, factors that have so often been ignored with respect to the residual, non-productive sections of the population.

This wider professional philosophy has remained largely undeveloped, certainly in the delivery of services to older people, and particularly in relation to health. Ageism has consistently lowered the priority older people receive, both in terms of resources, and the prestige associated with working with them. It is hoped that the new 'community care' legislation will assist in developing wider horizons in working with older people; certainly a more holistic approach can teach older people that good health consists of more than medical research, technology, drugs and professional health care.

THE PSYCHOLOGY OF MEDICAL AGEISM

A major objective of caring for older people should be to

overcome the impact of ageism, 'helping people to control their own ageing and to resist the social, environmental and health problems which can disrupt old age' (Phillipson and Strang, 1984). Many ageing people have low expectations about their health, and the access they have to professional support. These expectations can be reinforced by the activities and attitudes they experience from professional carers.

These problems require more acknowledgement in current professional intervention. The gratitude commonly shown by older people for whatever assistance they receive, regardless of whether it meets their needs, can lull carers into a false sense of their own value. Older people who require help often feel resentful, or fearful, about asking for it; others believe that nothing can be done. Indeed, given the ageist social climate in which decisions are reached, it is not always easy to see what remedies are available to ease the problems of social isolation and loneliness which accompany the ageing process (Black *et al.*, 1983). The result, as several studies have indicated, is that the psychological distress experienced by many older people can often be overlooked in social work assessments.

The expectations of older people are crucially important to the task of improving professional practice, and in overcoming resistance to change. For carers, helping older people should be about developing accurate self-awareness. Carers need to ascertain the assumptions upon which older people base their life, and provide them with information which challenges internalized social stereotypes, increases knowledge about the nature of the ageing process, and thereby raises personal expectations. Such information should assist older people to develop more positive outlooks, interpreting changes in health correctly, and emphasizing that ageing should be concerned with retaining rather than losing functioning abilities.

> Practitioners may be familiar with older persons who are depressed and immobilized by feelings about chronological age, even though functional capacities are undiminished, people whose expectations are too low or too high for their physical capacities, and those who persist in behaviours that are too physically or emotionally demanding because of their anxiety about appearing or feeling old. In such situations exploration and consideration with the client of his or her ideas and feelings about ageing may be helpful.
>
> (Furstenberg, 1989)

Convincing carers, and older people, that old age can be a positive experience, is crucial. Professional staff should seek to establish positive views about ageing by presenting images of older people as vital, joyful, able and attractive people. These can help older people to identify particular strengths that have been gained as the direct result of age, such as experience, a broader perspective, learned survival strategies and coping skills, The professional task is particularly important to older women, and older people from ethnic minority communities.

In considering the psychology of illness, the period following major loss or bereavement is often particularly perilous for older people. An important element of overcoming trauma is the individual's judgement that it can be overcome. Carers need to be particularly supportive at such times, exploring the person's attitudes, beliefs, anxieties and fears, helping the individual come to terms with the rest of his or her life by facilitating a more optimistic appraisal of what the future has to offer, and helping to plan activities that can assist him or her in regaining full functioning.

Counselling is a vital skill in combating negative attitudes to illness, and indicating to individuals what they can do for themselves (Scrutton, 1989). Maintaining optimism, and keeping faith with the body's ability to look after itself, via *vis medicatrix naturae*, is vital. The objective of self-help wherever possible and appropriate, must always remain uppermost in the professional task. Once this takes second place to giving help and assistance, older people are marginalized and reduced, both in our eyes, and in the eyes of the individual.

SOCIAL ISSUES

For professional intervention to be successful in dealing with the vital influence of social, economic, environmental and political factors on health, three distinct approaches are required. First, direct work with individuals should be aimed at maintaining and regenerating active personal involvement within the community, supporting individuals who enter old age with low self-esteem, and actively empowering the individual to take informed decisions about what constitutes a healthy lifestyle. The role of counselling when dealing with personality, gender and ethnic factors cannot be overemphasized (Scrutton, 1989). Sexual counselling can also prove to be invaluable.

The second arises from the need to tackle the ageism inherent within the society in which older people have to live.

Action in the broader environment is as important as intervention with individuals and groups. Social workers need to recognize the futility of activities to promote self-esteem when society denies the means for self-respect. Workers should attack the public sources of their clients' private troubles . . . (in order) . . . to create a social system that offers older people opportunities for remaining active and engaged.

(Furstenberg, 1989)

The third strand is to encourage the involvement of older people themselves in this wider, politicized social activity. Ultimately, this is perhaps the most useful contribution that younger carers can make, for to contest ageism *on behalf of older people* implicitly undermines the very arguments being made for them.

A number of activities can be organized which relate to the social aspects of healthy ageing. Carers can play a positive role in encouraging the formation of, and individual participation in, local groups. These groups can have a general purpose, concerned with discussing the ageing process, and stimulating physical and mental activity. Other groups can be educational, such as those dealing with issues of retirement; or therapeutic, such as counselling groups focusing on particular issues of concern. Support groups for family carers are also important, including self-help action groups for the carers of people with senile dementia, and other conditions. In dealing with group activities the particular needs of older women, and older people from ethnic minority communities, should always be considered.

Other groups can be aimed directly at health by combating loneliness and loss, dealing with specific issues such as depression and bereavement, providing counselling, and giving advice about relationships.

Dealing with issues relating to diet and nutrition are also best achieved through social involvement. Professional contact with older people includes the direct provision of meals, through meals-on-wheels, luncheon clubs, and residential care. Whilst this activity provides an opportunity to supply individuals with health-related diets, alongside nutritional information, such opportunities are usually neglected, apart from the simple notion of providing 'a balanced diet'. Even the provision of meals within hospital settings seldom pays attention to all the known aspects of healthy eating.

The impact of poor nutrition on health, and the role that professional counselling, advice, encouragement and education can play in relation to health, deserves attention, regardless of the setting in which contact with older people is made. Nutritionists, employed by local health authorities, can be usefully involved with individuals, or groups of older people. Professional involvement with older clients could then become less reactive to ageist perceptions, and more proactive in helping older people maintain their health through diet.

The existence of special diets for particular health problems is an area of work with individual people that has been almost totally neglected. The recognition of illnesses related to some form of food allergy or intolerance is also important. If there is no other identifiable cause of illness, such reactions can be investigated by the use of exclusion diets which can be developed without medical intervention. This approach is particularly useful in dealing with ailments such as migraine, asthma, colitis, and other chronic conditions. There are several steps that need to be taken:

1. Keep a detailed record of what is eaten.
2. Identify those foods and drinks (especially tea and coffee) for which there is a craving, or dependence.
3. Follow a diet which excludes these items, and which sticks to simple foods, like fruit and vegetables, recording food intake, and noting the impact on symptoms of illness.
4. Gradually expand the diet, item by item, identifying particular foods which bring back symptoms. This can be done by introducing single foods for several days, and taking nothing else but water, and noting the reaction.

If health does not improve, non-food allergies might requires investigation. This necessitates a thorough chemical clean-up, by identifying and removing all suspected chemicals used within the home. Doctors should be able to help commence a wider ecological investigation, or refer you to a clinical ecologist who can (Mackarness, 1980).

The physical aspects of good health should also be addressed, again through counselling, advice, encouragement and education. Encouraging exercise through groups can also be useful. In addition, the same non-medical help can be provided for older people who have problems relating to sleep, relaxation and posture.

One danger is that many carers over-care, and over-protect older people. It takes considerable skill to identify the real needs of an individual, and it is too easy to develop a 'false dependency' by supplying services which are simple to provide, but fail to address the underlying problem. The more tasks older people maintain for themselves, and the less physical support given, increases their physical activity, thereby helping to maintain their fitness and mobility.

The purpose of caring should be to encourage older people to retain their independence rather than undertaking tasks on their behalf, and to forestall the onset of disability rather than effecting a cure for health problems. Attention should focus on what can be done to prevent the ravages of ageing. In this, developing self-awareness about the origins of good health as something that lays in simple, self-help matters like social integration, good nutrition, and general fitness is important.

The development of local networks of caring professionals may help to create wider options for work with older people. Drawing together the sources of available help within the community may be able to stimulate more creative preventive strategies which encompass older people who are well, as well as those who are ill. Where there is inevitably a shortage of carers, individual work with older people can become depressing. Working alongside other people, who can bring with them different skills, perspectives and resources, is a way of avoiding this.

MEDICAL TREATMENT

In the event of illness, it is unnecessary to consider allopathic medicine as the first, or only, choice available. Carers should ensure that they are aware of the alternative options available within their areas by checking local press advertisements, the 'yellow pages' of the telephone directory, or writing for local information from the national organizations listed in the directory (Appendix).

In large urban areas, health centres are now being established which offer a wide variety of alternative therapies. There are also increasing demands to establish information and counselling services within mainstream medical centres and hospitals. Whilst most alternative medicine remains outside the National Health Service, some doctors are beginning to use other forms of medicine, particularly homeopathy, and this might be available locally. The trend towards wider choice is likely to grow. At the time of writing, the policy of the Labour Party is to include alternative therapy within the National Health Service.

There is a need for carers to develop more open, enquiring approaches, to develop, extend and broaden their knowledge base, particularly in being more aware when alternative methods can be used. The prevalent idea seems to be that alternative approaches should be sought after allopathic medicine has failed. This is probably wrong, particularly if the homeopathic concept of working alongside the body, and the naturopathic philosophy that repressing acute illness leads to chronic disease, are considered. Indeed, many alternative approaches, particularly the sensory, manipulative and exercise therapies, are probably best used as preventative rather than as curative medical techniques.

AN APPROACH TO DEATH

There is a strong need for an open approach to personal loss, bereavement and death. In particular, there is a need to reach a balance between living life realistically to the full, and maintaining an open acceptance of the inevitability of death.

It is difficult for many carers to assist ageing people in this way, principally because few people in Western society have such an attitude themselves. How helpful carers can be without spending time examining our own attitudes and feelings about loss, and death, is uncertain. Perhaps, more than any other area of training for those working with older people, this is vital.

To give genuine assistance within the mourning process, to counsel grief and bereavement, and to guide the older individual towards personal death, is a difficult procedure, both in terms of the skills, personal empathy, and the understanding of the processes involved. There are also moral and religious attitudes, as well as medical attitudes that have to be considered. Carers have to be aware of their personal attitudes towards, for example, euthanasia, not just as a philosophical issue, but as a practical matter if and when confronted with it. This will need to be closely linked with personal attitudes towards medical efforts to prolong life and to prevent death.

Opportunities for this can be taken by openly discussing with older people the death of acquaintances, pets, or people in the news. It is important, however, to recognize that such discussion can be emotionally distressing, and it is always advisable for carers to seek to share their personal difficulties with colleagues or friends who are capable of playing the role of the counsellor's counsellor.

Skills have been developed in working with bereavement and death. Those working in bereavement counselling, and in the hospice movement are notable. More general skills, including reminiscence and life-story work, can help to make sense of the life that is ending, for everyone concerned. It is important that carers face the challenges that death presents, and that there is no attempt to postpone discussing the subject, or discussing it morbidly. The best advice for older people is probably to plan their life as if they had another 10, 20 or 30 years to live, whilst living each day on the assumption that it might be their last. The best advice for the carer is to encourage older people to do just this.

When serious illness brings closer the prospect of death, it is important that honesty is maintained. It is still not necessary to accept the inevitability of death 'today', but to recognize and come to terms with the likelihood of death 'tomorrow'. The best advice remains to continue cherishing each day without destroying it with fear, and to make all the necessary preparations, including perhaps, making a 'living will' which states their wishes if illness or disablement strikes short of death, whilst time remains.

CONCLUSION

The issue of health in old age needs to be recontextualized and demedicalized. The aim should be not to prevent old age, or even delay death, but to maintain the quality of life until closer to death whilst, at the same time, to help older people come to terms with death. The recontextualizing of elderly health is possible if four objectives are pursued:

1. *Confronting the ageism which makes the prospect and experience of old age so depressing.* Many of the problems of old age are socially constructed, arising from the way older people are expected to live within the confines of the social status attributed to those who have lost their productive and nurturing roles, and the economic status granted to them by subsistence pensions. If old age is depressing it is because it has been made so; the solution does not lie with a prescription for anti-depressants.

2. *Challenging the dominant assumptions about health and old age, especially those concerning the origins of ill health.* Medical ageism has to be tackled. Ill health is not a natural, or inevitable consequence of old age, but the belief that it is represents the single, most important reason for the low priority of elderly care.

3. *Reaffirming individual control over health.* The social construction of old age indicates that many solutions lay within social structures in which the individual can exercise some control. There are many factors which contribute to health, many under the direct control of the older individual. Illich (1977) argued

that the layman, not the physician, has the perspective, and the power to stop the iatrogenesis of allopathic medicine.

4. *Increasing individual awareness of good health, giving knowledge of the methods and techniques available, and how good health can be achieved and maintained.* Reasserting personal control is impossible without adequate knowledge. The 'de-skilling' of the ageing individual, and their carers, has to be reversed by a process that can be started if people are aware of their potential role, and the role that can be played by alternative medical practitioners.

When these factors are taken into consideration, the impact of medicine on the health of older people assumes a different perspective. Yet, whilst medicine spends vast sums each year on attempts to discover 'mechanical' medical answers to the problems of disease, with increasingly more complicated machinery, heroic operations, expensive and dangerous drugs, the potential role that professional carers can play in the prevention of ill health needs to be increasingly recognized.

Useful addresses

DIRECTORY OF USEFUL ADDRESSES

General

Age Concern
Astral House
1268 London Road
London SW16 4ER

Help the Aged
1 Sekforde Street
London EC1

Centre for Policy on Ageing
25–31 Ironmonger Row
London EC1V 3QP

Christian Council on Ageing
The Old Court
Greens Norton
Nr Towcester
Northants NN12 8BS

Self-help groups

Pensioners' Protection Party
PO Box 5
Torquay
Devon

Association of Retired Persons
Borough Woods House
Shillingford
Nr. Bampton
Devon EX16 9BL

Pensioners' Rights Campaign
2 Harlington Place
Carlisle
Cumbria CA1 1HL

Pensioners' Liaison Forum
398 Simpson Village
Bletchley
Milton Keynes MK6 3AL

Pensioners' Voice
Melling House
91 Preston New Road
Blackburn BB2 6BD

British Pensioners/Trades Union Action Association
87 Kings Drive
Gravesend
Kent DA12 5BQ

Support groups

Carer's National Association
29 Chilworth Mews
London W2 3RG

Pre-Retirement Association
19 Undine Street
Tooting
London SW17 8PP

Conference of Ethnic Minority Senior Citizens
5–5a Westminster Bridge Road
London SE1 7SW

Depressives Associated
PO Box 5
Castletown
Portland
Dorset DT5 1BQ

Gay Men's Disabled Group
c/c Gay's the Word Bookshop
66 Marchmont Street
London WC1N 1AB

GEMMA (Lesbians with/without disabilities)
PO Box 5700
London WC1N 3XX

National Association of Widows
54–57 Allison Street
Digbeth
Birmingham B5 5TH

National Council for Divorced, Separated
13 High Street
Little Shelford
Cambridgeshire CB2 5ES

Women's Health and Reproductive Rights
52–54 Featherstone Street
London EC1Y 8RT

Counselling

British Association for Counselling
37a Sheep Street
Rugby CV21 3BX

CRUSE – Bereavement Care
Cruse House
126 Sheen Road
Richmond
Surrey TW9 1UR

Relate (National Marriage Guidance)
Herbert Gray College
Rugby
Warwickshire CV21 3AP

Education

National Institute of Adult Education
19B De Montford Street
Leicester LE1 7GE

Workers Educational Association
9 Upper Berkeley Street
London W1

Open University
Admissions office
PO Box 48
Milton Keynes MK7 6AA

Alternative medicine

Institute for Complementary Medicine
21 Portland Place
London W1N 3AF

or

Suite 1
19a Cavendish Square
London W1N 9A

Alternative Action
Carlton House
11 Marlborough Place
Brighton
East Sussex NN1 1UB

Health Information Centre
Green House
Bangor
Gwynedd LL57 1AX

British Holistic Medical Association
179 Gloucester Place
London NW1 6DX

Natural Medicines Society
95 Hagley Road
Edgbaston
Birmingham B16 8LA

Naturopathy and osteopathy

British Naturopathic/Osteopathic Association
Frazer House
6 Netherhall Gardens
London NW3 5RR

General Council and Register of Osteopaths
21 (or 1–4) Suffolk Street
London SW1Y 4HG

Homeopathy

British Homoeopathic Association
27a Devonshire Street
London W1N 1RJ

Society of Homoeopaths
2a Bedford Place
Southampton
Hampshire SO1 2BY

or

47 Canada Grove
Bognor Regis
West Sussex PO21 1DW

Herbalism

National Institute of Medical Herbalists
41 Hatherley Road
Winchester
Hampshire SO22 6RR

School of Herbal Medicine
Bucksteep Manor
Bodle Street Green
Hailsham BN27 4RJ

Dr Christopher School of Natural Healing
19 Park Terrace
Stoke-on-Trent
Staffordshire

School of Natural Medicine
Dolphin House
6 Gold Street
Saffron Waldon
Essex CB10 1EJ

British Herbal Medicine Association
The Old Coach House
Southborough Road
Surbiton
Surrey

General Council/Register of Consultant Herbalists
Marlborough House
Swanpool
Falmouth
Cornwall TR11 4HW

Acupuncture

The British Acupuncture Association
34 Alderney Street
London SW1V 4EU

Traditional Acupuncture Society
11 Grange Park
Stratford-upon-Avon
Warwickshire CV37 6XH

Registrar of Traditional Chinese Medicine
7a Thorndean Street
London SW18 4HE

The Council for Acupuncture
19a Cavendish Square
London W1M 9AD

Yoga

British Wheel of Yoga
1 Hamilton Place
Boston Road
Sleaford
Lincolnshire

or

15 Station Avenue
Warwick CV34 5HJ

Yoga for Health Foundation
Ickwell Bury
Northill
Biggleswade
Bedfordshire SG18 9ES

Reflexology

British Reflexology Association
12 Pond Road
London SE3 9JL

Bayly School of Reflexology Ltd
Monks Orchard
Whitbourne
Worcester WR6 5RB

Exercise

Extend
5 Conway Road
Sheringham
Norfolk NR26 8DD

Relaxation for Living
29 Burwood Park Road
Walton-on-Thames
Surrey KT12 5LH

Cancer

New Approaches to Cancer
c/o The Seekers Trust
Addington Park
Maidstone
Kent ME19 5BL

BACUP (British Association of Cancer United Patients)
121/123 Charterhouse Street
London EC1M 6AA

Cancer Help Centre
Grove House
Cornwallis Grove
Clifton
Bristol BS8 4PG

Cancerlink
17 Britannia Street
London WC1X 9JN

Hearing

Royal National Institute for Deaf
105 Gower Street
London WC1E 6AH

British Association of Hard of Hearing
6 Great James Street
London WC1N 3DA

Sight

Royal National Institute for Blind
224 Great Portland Street
London W1N 6AA

Disability sexuality

SPOD (Association to aid sexual, personal relationships of people with disability)
286 Camden Road
London N7 0BJ

Association of Sexual, Marital Therapists
PO Box 62
Sheffield S10 3TS

General illnesses

Alzheimer's Disease Society
158–160 Balham High Road
London SW12 9BN

Arthritis Care
5 Grosvenor Crescent
London SW1X 7ER

Breast Care and Mastectomy Association
26a Harrison Street
London WC1H 8JG

Chest, Heart and Stroke Association
Tavistock House North
Tavistock Square
London WC1H 9JE

Colostomy Welfare Group
38–39 Eccleston Square
London SW1V 1PB

National Osteoporosis Society
PO Box 10
Barton Meade House
Radstock
Bath
Avon BA3 3YB

Parkinson's Disease Society
36 Portland Place
London W1N 3DG

Alexander technique

Society of Teachers of Alexander Technique
London House
26b Fulham Road
London SW10 9EL

References

Adler, William H., Jones, Kenneth H. and Brock, Mary Anne (1978) Aging and immune function, in *Biology of Aging* (eds Behnke, John A., Finch, Caleb E. and Moment, Gairdner, B.) Pelum Press, New York.

Argyle, Michael (1987) *The Psychology of Happiness*. Methuen, London.

Aries, P. (1983) *The Hour of Our Death*, Peregrine, London.

Ashton, David and Davies, Bruce (1986) *Why Exercise? Expert Medical Advice to Help you Enjoy a Healthier Life*, Basil Blackwell, Oxford.

Asplund, K., Normark M. and Pettersson, V. (1981) Nutritional assessment of psychogeriatric patients. *Age and Ageing*. **10**.

Beauvoir, Simone de (1966) *A Very Easy Death*, Andre Deutsch and George Weidenfeld, London.

Beauvoir, Simone de (1972) *Old Age*, Deutsch, Wiedenfeld and Nicholson, London.

Benjamin, Harry (1936, 1961) *Everybody's Guide to Nature Cure*, Thorsons, Wellingborough.

Bhadura, Reba (1989) A prescription for counselling. *Social Work Today*, 30 November.

Black, J. et al., (1983) *Social Work in Context*. Tavistock, London.

Blair, Pat (1985) *Know Your Medicines*, Age Concern England, London.

Bohm, David (1981) *Wholeness and the Implicate Order*, Routledge & Kegan Paul, London.

Bowling, A. and Cartwright, A. (1982) *Life After a Death: a Study of the Elderly Widowed*, Tavistock, London.

British Social Attitudes (1987) Gower, Aldershot.

Brown, Margaret (1988) *Keep Moving, Keep Young: Gentle Yoga Exercises for the Elderly*, Unwin, London.

Cailliet, Rene and Gross, Leonard (1987) *Growing Young: the Fitness Strategy to Reverse the Effects of Ageing*, Grafton Books, London.

Caine, Lynne (1975) *Widow*, Macdonald and Janes, London.

Cannon, Geoffrey (1989) *The Good Fight: the Life and Work of Caroline Walker*, Ebury, London.

Capra, Fritjof (1975) *The Tao of Physics*, Wildwood House, Aldershot.

Carlson, Rick J. (1975) *The Frontiers of Science and Medicine*, Wildwood House, Aldershot.

'Ceres' (1984) *The Healing Power of Herbal Teas*, Thorsons, Wellingborough.

Chaitow, Leon (1990) *Osteopathic Self-treatment: Safe and Effective Self-help Techniques for Relaxing Tense Muscles and Easing Pain*, Thorsons, Wellingborough.

Cheraskin, E., Ringsdorg, W.M. and Brecher, Arline (1974) *Psychodietetics: Food as the Key to Emotional Health*, Stein and Day, New York.

Cochrane, A.L. (1972) *Effectiveness and Efficiency*, The Nuffield Provincial Hospitals Trust, London.

Coleman, Vernon (1986a) *Natural Pain Control*, Century Arrow, London.

Coleman, Vernon (1986b) *Mind Power – How to Use Your Mind to Heal Your Body*, Century, London.

Comfort, Alex (1977) *A Good Age*, Mitchell Beazley, London.

Cousins, Norman (1979) *Anatomy of an Illness as Perceived by The Patient: Reflections on Healing and Regeneration*, Norton, New York.

Cummings, E. and Henry, W.E. (1961) *Growing Old: the Process of Disengagement*, Basic Books, New York.

Donovan, J. (1986) *We Don't Buy Sickness, It Just Comes*, Gower, Aldershot.

Doyle, Leslie (1983) *The Political Economy of Health*, Pluto, London.

Dubos, Rene (1959) *Mirage and Health: Utopias, Progress and Biological Change*, George Allen & Unwin, London.

Dubos, Rene (1970) *Man, Medicine and Environment*, Penguin, Harmondsworth.

Eckardt, Michael J. (1978) Consequences of alcohol and other drug use in aged, in *Biology of Aging* (eds Behnke, John A., Finch, Caleb E. and Moment, Gairdner, B.) Pelum Press, New York.

Ehrenreich, Barbara, and English, Dierdre (1973) *Complaints and Disorders: the Sexual Politics of Sickness*, Writers and Readers Co-operative, London.

Evers, H. (1985) The frail elderly woman: emergent questions in ageing and women's health, *Women, Health and Healing: Towards a New Perspective*, (eds Lewin, E. and Olesen, V.), Tavistock, London.

Exton-Smith, A.N. (1971) Nutrition and the elderly. *British Journal of Hospital Medicine*, May, 639–46.

Fennel, Graham, Phillipson, Chris and Evers, Helen (1988) *The Sociology of Old Age*, Open University Press, Milton Keynes.

Finch, J. and Groves, D. (1982) By women for women: caring for the frail elderly. *Women's Studies International Forum*, **5**.

Freud, S.(1905) *On Psychotherapy*, Hogarth Press, London.

Friedman, Meyer and Ulmer, Diane (1985) *Treating Type A Behaviour and Your Heart*, Michael Joseph, London.

Fromm, Erich (1957) *The Art of Loving*, Allen and Unwin, London.

Fulder, Stephen (1983) *An End to Ageing: Traditional and Modern Ways of Extending Healthy Life*, Thorsons, Wellingborough.

Fulder, Stephen (1988) *The Handbook of Complementary Medicine*, 2nd edn, Oxford University Press, Oxford.

Furstenberg, Anna-Linda (1989) Older people's age self-concept. Social Casework. *Journal of Contemporary Social Work*, May.

Furth, Anna and Harding, John (1989) Why sugar is bad for you. *New Scientist*, 23 September.

Georgakas, Dan (1980) *The Methuselah Factors: the Secrets of the World's Longest Lived Peoples*, Simon and Schuster, New York.

Gidley, Isobelle and Shears, Richard (1988) *Alzheimer's: What it is, How to Cope*, Unwin Hyman, London.

Glaser, B. and Strauss, A. (1965) *Awareness of Dying*, Weidenfeld and Nicholson, London.

Goldberg, E.M. and Connelly, N. (1982) *The Effectiveness of Social Care for the Elderly*, Heinemann/PSI, London.

Gore, Irene (1973) *Age and Vitality: Commonsense Ways of Adding Life to Your Years*, Allen and Unwin, London.

Graham, Margaret (1988) *Keep Moving, Keep Young: Gentle Exercises for the Elderly*, Unwin, London.

Greengross, Wendy and Greengross, Sally (1989) *Living, Loving and Ageing: Sexual and Personal Relationships in Later Life*, Age Concern England, London.

Griggs, Barbara (1981) *Green Pharmacy: a History of Herbal Medicine*, Robert Hale, London.

Hills, Margaret (1985) *Curing Arthritis: the Drug-free Way*, Sheldon, London.

Hite, Shere (1977) *The Hite Report: a Nationwide Study of Female Sexuality*, Collier Macmillan, London.

Hodgkinson, Liz (1987) *Smile Therapy*. Optima, London.

Hoffman, David (1983) *The Holistic Herbal: a Herbal Celebrating the Wholeness of Life*, Findhorn Press, Moray.

Hoffman, David (1986) *Herbal Stress Control*, Thorsons, Wellingborough.

Hoffman, David (1990) *The Elements of Herbalism*, Element Books, Shaftesbury.,

Hope, Murray (1989) *The Psychology of Healing*, Element Books, Shaftesbury.

Hunt, E.H. (1990) Paupers and pensioners: past and present, *Ageing and Society*, **9**.

Hunt, Teresa (1988) *Growing Older, Living Longer: Revolutionary Breakthroughs in the Science of Ageing*, Bodley Head, London.

Hurwitz, Natalie and Wade, O.L. (1969) Intensive hospital monitoring of adverse reactions to drugs. *British Medical Journal*, **1**, 531–6.

Illich, Ivan (1977) *Limits to Medicine: Medical Nemesis; the Expropriation of Health*, Penguin, Harmondsworth.

Inglis, Brian and West, Ruth (1983) *The Alternative Health Guide*, Michael Joseph, London.

Jackson, Judith (1986) *Aromatherapy*, Dorling Kindersley, London.

Jones, Chris (1983) *State Social Work and the Working Class*, Macmillan, London.

Kent, Howard (1985) *Yoga for the Disabled; a Practical Self-Help Guide to a Happier Healthier Life*, Thorsons, Wellingborough.

Kenyon, Julian (1987) *Acupressure Technique: a Self-help Guide: Home Treatment for a Wide Range of Conditions*, Thorsons, Wellingborough.

Kidman, Brenda (1983) *A Gentle Way with Cancer: What Every Cancer Patient Should Know About the Therapies Which Can Influence the Fight for Recovery*, Century, London.

Kohli, Martin (1988) Ageing as a challenge for sociological theory. *Ageing and Society*, **8**.

Kubler-Ross, E. (1973) *On Death and Dying*, Tavistock, London.

Lamy, P.L. (1981) Nutrition and the elderly. *Drug Intelligence and Clinical Pharmacy*, **15** (Nov).

Levin, Lowell, S., Katz, Alfred, H. and Holst, Eric (1977) *Self-care: Lay Initiatives in Health*, Croom Helm, London.

Lovelock, J.E. (1979) *Gaia: a New Look at Life on Earth*, Oxford University Press, Oxford.

McEwen, Evelyn (1990) *Age: the Unrecognised Discrimination: Views to Provoke a Debate*, Age Concern England, London.

McIntyre, Anne (1987), *Herbal Medicine*, McDonald Optima, London.

Mackarness, Richard (1976) *Not All in the Mind*, Pan, London.

Mackarness, Richard (1980) *Chemical Victims*, Pan, London.

McKeown, Thomas (ed) (1979) *The Role of Medicine: Dream, Mirage or Nemesis?* Blackwell, Oxford.

Mansfield, Peter (1988) *The Good Health Book: Help Yourself Get Better*, Grafton Books, London.

Masters, William H. and Johnson, Virginia E. (1966) *Human Sexual Response*, Little, Brown, Boston.

Meade, K. (1986) *Age Well Campaign: Challenging the Myths: a Campaign to Promote Health activities for and with Older People*, Pensioners Link, Barnet, Health Education Project (with Health Education Council and Age Concern), London.

Minois, Georges (1989) *History of Old Age*. Polity Press, Cambridge.

Mitchell, Jeannette (1984) *What is to be Done About Illness and Health?* Penguin, Harmondsworth.

Monsour, N. and Robb, S. (1982) Wandering behaviour in old age: a psychological study. *Social Work*, Sept.

Neugarten, Bernice (ed) (1969) *Middle Age and Ageing*, University of Chicago Press, Chicago.

Norman, Allison (1985) *Triple Jeopardy: Growing Old in a Second Homeland*, Centre for Policy on Ageing, London.

Norman, Allison (1987) *Aspects of Ageism: a Discussion Paper*, Centre for Policy on Ageing, London.

Ornstein, Robert E. and Sobel, David (1988) *The Healing Brain: a Radical New Approach to Health Care*, Macmillan, London.

Parkes, C.M. (1972) *Bereavement: Studies of Grief in Adult Life*, Tavistock, London.

Parsons, Talcott (1970) *The Social System*, Routledge and Kegan Paul, London.

Passwater, Richard A. (1986) *Cancer and its Nutritional Therapies*, Keats, Horsham.

Pelletier, Kenneth R. (1978) *Mind as Healer; Mind as Slayer: a Holistic Approach to Preventing Stress Disorders*, Allen and Unwin, London.

Phillips, David A. (1983) *New Dimensions in Health: from Soil to Psyche*, Angus & Robertson, Sydney.

Phillipson, Chris and Strang, Patricia (1984) *Health Education and Older People: the Role of Paid Carers*, Health Education Council, University of Keele.

Phillipson, Chris and Strang, Patricia (1986) *Training and Education for an Ageing Society: New Perspectives for the Health and Social Services*, Health Education Council, University of Keele.

Posner, B.M. (1979) *Nutrition and the Elderly*, Lexington Books, Massachusetts.

Richard, Dick (1982) *The Topic of Cancer: When the Killing Has to Stop*, Pergamon, Oxford.

Runcie, J. (1981) Nutritional problems in the elderly. *The Practitioner*, Dec., pp. 1747–52.

Schauss, Alexander (1985) *Nutrition and Behaviour*, Keats, New Canaan, Connecticut.

Schorah, C.J. and Morgan, D.B. (1985) Nutritional deficiencies in the elderly. *Hospital Update*, May.

Scrutton, Steve (1989) *Counselling Older People: a Creative Response to Ageing*, Age Concern England/Edward Arnold, London.

Scrutton, Steve (1990) Ageism: the basis of age discrimination, in Age: the Unrecognised Discrimination: Views to Provoked Debate, (ed Evelyn McEwen), Age Concern England, London.

Selye, Hans (1956) *The Stress of Life*, McGraw Hill, New York.

Sheldrake, Rupert (1987) *A New Science of Life: Hypothesis at Formative Causation*, Paladin, London.

Shreeve, Caroline M. (1986) *The Alternative Dictionary of Symptoms and Cures: a Comprehensive Guide to Diseases and their Orthodox and Alternative Remedies*, Century, London.

Smith, Trevor (1982) *Homeopathic Medicine: a Doctor's Guide to Remedies for Common Ailments*, Thorsons, Wellingborough.

Sontag, S. (1973) *Illness as Metaphor*, Penguin, Harmondsworth.

Stanway, Andrew (1982) *Alternative Medicine: a Guide to Natural Therapies*, Penguin, Harmondsworth.

Starr, B.D. and Bakur-Weiner, M. (1982) *The Starr-Weiner Report on Sex and Sexuality in the Mature Years*, McGraw-Hill, New York.

Stoppard, Miriam (1983) *50+ Lifeguard: How to Ensure Fitness, Health and Happiness in the Middle Years and Beyond*. Dorling Kindersley, London.

Straten, Michael van (1987) *The Complete Natural Health Consultant*, Ebury Press, London.

Thunhurst, Colin (1982) *It Makes you Sick: the Politics of the NHS*, Pluto, London.

Thompson, D. (1984) The decline of social welfare: falling state suport for the elderly since Victorian times. Ageing and Society, **4**.

Trattler, Ross (1985) *Better Health Through Natural Healing: How to Get Well Without Drugs or Surgery*, Thorsons, Wellingborough.

Tyler, W. (1986) Structural ageism as a phenomenon in British society. *Journal of Education Gerontology*. Keele.

Viorst, Judith (1986) *Necessary Losses: the Loves, Illusions, Dependencies and Impossible Expectations that all of us Have to Give Up in Order to Grow*, Simon & Schuster, London.

Walford, Roy L. (1983) *Maximum Life-span*. W.W. Norton, New York.

Walker, A. (1983) Care for elderly people: a conflict between women and the state, in A Labour of Love: Women, Work and Caring (eds J. Finch and D. Groves), Routledge and Kegan Paul, London.

Watson, George (1972) *Nutrition and Your Mind: the Psychochemical Response*, Harper and Row, London.

Weber, Max (1930) *The Protestant Ethic and the Spirit of Capitalism*, Allen and Unwin, London.

Whitehead, Margaret, Townsend, Peter and Davison, Nick (1988) *Inequalities of Health: the Black Report, and The Health Divide*, Penguin, Harmondsworth.

Williamson, J. and Chopin, Joan M. (1980) Adverse reactions to prescribed drugs in the elderly: a multicentre investigation. *Age and Ageing*, **19** (2).

Wurtman, Judith (1988) *Managing your Mind and Mood Through Food*, Grafton, London.

Younghusband, E. (1951) *Social Work in Britain: a Supplementary Report on Employment and Training of Social Workers*, Constable, Edinburgh.

Younghusband, E. (1978) *Social Work in Britain, 1950–1975*, Allen and Unwin, London.

Index